THE ADOLESCENT SPINE

MODERN ORTHOPEDIC MONOGRAPHS

Series Consultant

Robert E. Leach, M.D.
Boston University School of Medicine

THE ADOLESCENT SPINE

HUGO A. KEIM, M.D., F.A.C.S.

*Associate Clinical Professor of Orthopaedic
Surgery, College of Physicians and Surgeons,
Columbia University, New York; Associate
Attending Orthopaedic Surgeon and Chief,
Scoliosis Service, New York Orthopaedic Hospital,
Columbia-Presbyterian Medical Center, New York;
Attending Orthopaedic Surgeon and Chief,
Scoliosis Clinic, Helen Hayes Hospital,
West Haverstraw, New York; Attending Orthopaedic
Surgeon, Francis Delafield Hospital, New York;
Consulting Orthopaedic Surgeon, Holy Name Hospital,
Teaneck, New Jersey*

GRUNE & STRATTON
A Subsidiary of Harcourt Brace Jovanovich, Publishers

New York   San Francisco   London

Library of Congress Cataloging in Publication Data

Keim, Hugo A
    The adolescent spine.

    (Modern orthopedic monographs)
    Bibliography
    Includes index.
    1. Spine—Diseases. 2. Spine—Abnormities and
deformities. 3. Youth—Diseases. I. Title.
(DNIM: 1. Spinal diseases—In adolescence. WE725
K27a)
RJ480.K38   617'.375   75-32566
ISBN 0-8089-0923-1

Grune & Stratton, Inc.
111 Fifth Avenue
New York, New York 10003

Library of Congress Catalog Card Number 75-32566
International Standard Book Number 0-8089-0923-1
Printed in the United States of America

TO MY MOTHER AND FATHER

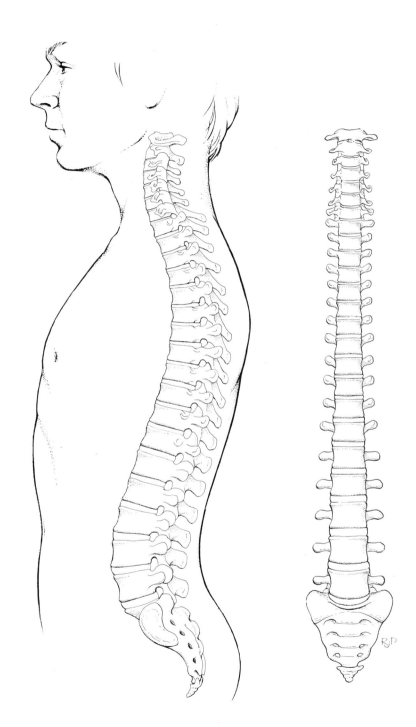

CONTENTS

INTRODUCTION

As the population of the world continues to grow, and as the lifespan of man increases with the help of modern science and medical technology, the human skeleton is required to function for longer periods of time. Many problems that besiege the adult in relation to the skeletal system come from abnormalities that exist during infantile and adolescent periods. These can be in the form of congenital problems at birth or situations acquired due to environment or trauma. We all know that an automobile which is driven for a long period of time tends to show its wear and tear by rust and rattles. The human frame, if abused during the important adolescent years, will show these effects with pains and disabilities in the adult, especially during the so-called "golden" period of a person's life.

A book on the adolescent spine is considered to be pertinent at this time because so little "living anatomy" is taught in medical schools. Adolescents today are much more active and are subjected to an infinite array of traumatizing episodes in the form of sports and hobbies which make them prone to all kinds of injuries and diseases. It is hoped that this book, by starting with the embryological and anatomical basics of the human spine, and applying them to the physical findings in the treatment of youngsters with spinal problems, will help to elucidate the confusing picture of spinal conditions between the child and adult. Many times children are extremely well cared for by pediatricians, but somehow fall into a gap created between the pediatric age group and adulthood. There is a need for physicians interested specifically in the orthopedic problems of the adolescent, since so many important situations and difficult problems arise during this phase of life.

Knowledge about the human spine is increasing at a rather rapid pace. However, new knowledge either extends or outmodes the old. It forces us to relearn today what we thought we knew yesterday, and has led Dr. Robert Hilliard, of the Federal Communications Commission, to state "At the rate at which knowledge is growing, by the time a child born today graduates from college, the amount of knowledge in the world will be four times as great. By the time that same child is fifty years old, it will be thirty-two times as great, and 97% of everything known in the world will have been learned since the time he was born."[1] Since we are becoming overwhelmed with new material for absorption every day of our lives, we must make changes and apply what

1. Toffler A: Future Shock (ed 1). London, Pan Books Ltd, 1973, p 149

modern technology and applied science has found out for us. Basic anatomy never changes; however applied science, in the treatment of pathological disturbances of this anatomy, has been in constant change since the time of Hippocrates.

It is my fond hope this book will in some way help to shed some light on the adolescent spine and the problems of spinal diagnosis and treatment during a very complicated and volatile period in a person's life. All medical teachers like to think that they have left their mark in some way on their students, so that the knowledge they may have imparted will be passed on to improve the care and management of people afflicted with medical problems. The knowledge that many of the young men and women whom I have been privileged to teach will be going out into practice to impart some of these principles has already been my reward. Hopefully, this book will serve the same purpose for students who will read it.

I would like to express my thanks to the many educators and former teachers who have helped me to formulate some of the basic facts as I understand them. Particularly Dr. Frank E. Stinchfield, my Chief at the New York Orthopaedic Hospital of the Columbia-Presbyterian Medical Center, for his unselfish devotion and dedication to helping residents and young staff members. His constant encouragement and advice have been invaluable. I would also like to thank many other physicians, teachers, and friends who have been a great source of help to me and are too numerous to mention individually.

To my wife, Ruth, and Sharon, Steven, Paula, and Gregory, thank you for your love and understanding during long hours that I have been unable to share with you.

FOREWORD

It is my great privilege to contribute a foreward to this excellent book —The Adolescent Spine. The book, which is a comprehensive work on adolescent spinal problems, clearly reflects the author's wide clinical experience.

Dr. Keim, at a young age, has limited his work to the study and treatment of the human spine—not only in the clinical field but in research as well. He has immersed himself thoroughly in all aspects of this subject. The material is clearly and authoritatively presented. It is a scholarly text, carefully organized, with each chapter containing valuable information on the area covered. I believe that medical students, residents, and experienced orthopaedic surgeons all will derive benefits and valuable assistance from this book.

Among the outstanding features are the photographs, x-ray reproductions, and excellent art work of Mr. Robert Demerest.

The New York Orthopaedic Hospital, of the Columbia-Presbyterian Medical Center, in which Dr. Keim is doing his work, has always been recognized for its orthopaedic surgeons who have made the spine their particular specialty. The author has been a worthy successor to such men as Doctors Russell Hibbs, Joseph Risser, William H. Von Lackum, and Theodore Waugh, all of whom preceded him in this specialized field.

Dr. Keim has always been an enthusiastic teacher of orthopaedic surgery, especially in the field of scoliosis. He was done a remarkable job in writing this book which I believe will stand the test of time. I recommend the book to the physician who is looking for advice on how to diagnose and treat the adolescent patient with a spinal problem. I found the text interesting, informative, instructive, and highly readable. Dr. Keim is to be complimented.

Frank E. Stinchfield, M.D.

ACKNOWLEDGMENTS

It has often been said that every person has at least one novel or textbook inside of him. Here is my offering; hopefully my efforts will be appreciated and rewarded by the students who read this work. I would like to acknowledge, however, that in writing a book of this kind there are many people behind the scenes who do not receive the credit that they should, but who are extremely important in the formation and execution of the material which goes to complete the finished product. I would like to thank Mr. Robert J. Demerest for his excellent art work throughout the entire text. He is a very gifted artist in the medical world and has won numerous awards attesting to his many skills. It was an extreme pleasure and privilege to be able to work with him on the illustrations and also to be able to appreciate the hard work that goes into the artistic creation of an idea or theme.

My book secretary, Ms. Kathy Bailey, has been an invaluable assistant to me, not only during times of mental lapse and depression, but during times of sporadic elation when she had a levelling effect and constantly helped to put together many rambling thoughts which I had into a coherent and grammatically acceptable form. She accomplished her task while also working toward her Ph.D. and managing her family. I am most appreciative of her unselfish efforts.

Mr. William Humphrey of the Deering-Milliken Corporation has been most encouraging and helpful during the past six years in urging me to put my thoughts on paper. The financial assistance of Mr. Roger Milliken and the Deering-Milliken Corporation has been greatly appreciated in helping to defray the many expenses of writing a book in these inflationary times.

Finally, I would like to thank Grune & Stratton for the tremendous aid and encouragement in helping me bring this effort to press.

Hugo A. Keim, M.D.
January, 1976

THE ADOLESCENT SPINE

1

Embryology and Anatomy of the Human Spine

The development of the human spine is a very rapid embryological phenomenon. During a few brief weeks, the entire anatomical pattern of a lifetime of spinal stability or abnormality is established.

We sometimes fail to realize that infants are not little children, and that children are not small adults. There are many differences between the spines of the infant, child, adolescent, and adult, which cause the spine and its contents to be vulnerable to a myriad of individual and specific problems at each stage of spinal development and growth.

The embryological development of the human spine can be divided into four concurrent stages that blend into each other. The first stage, the notochord stage, starts at about the 15th day of life and persists with remnants into adulthood. The second stage of spinal development is the membranous stage, which begins at about 21 days and ends during the 3rd month of gestation. The third stage, the cartilage stage, begins at 5 to 6 weeks and continues throughout fetal life. The fourth and final stage is the bony stage, which begins during the 2nd month of life but is only partially complete at birth (Fig. 1-1).

Many developmental aberrations can produce congenital anomalies during any of the four stages. Aberrations are common during the membranous stage, when the mesenchyme starts to form around the notochord. Once this mold or precursor pattern is established, the cartilage and bony stages merely follow the established deformity, so that at birth the anomaly is almost fully developed and can be quite severe.

Between the 14th and 21st days in the development of an embryo, the amniotic cavity and the yolk sac are separated by a platelike layer of cells that

1

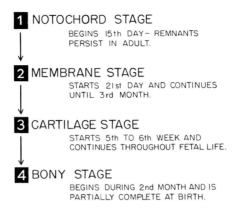

Fig. 1-1.   Four stages of embryonic and fetal development.

have already begun to divide into the ectoderm, mesoderm, and endoderm. The neural plate develops from the ectoderm and later flexes to form the neural groove and subsequently the neural tube. (Fig. 1-2)

Along the sides of the neural tube, the cells of the mesodermal germ layer form a thin sheet of loosely woven connective tissue. By about the 17th day, some of these cells close to the midline proliferate and form a thickened plate of tissue known as the dorsal mesoderm (Fig. 1-2A). More laterally, the mesoderm layer remains thin and is known as the lateral mesoderm. These two mesodermal layers are connected by the same type of tissue, and this is termed the intermediate mesoderm. Near the midline, the mesodermal tissue coalesces and forms the somite from the previously formed dorsal mesoderm. With the appearance of the lateral plate, an intracellular cavity develops to separate the plate and divide the tissue into two layers (Fig. 1-2B): (1) a layer continuous with the extra-embryonic mesoderm covering the amnion, known as the somatic, or parietal, mesoderm layer; and (2) a layer continuous with the mesoderm covering the yolk sac, known as the splanchnic, or visceral, mesoderm layer.

The notochord lies just beneath the neural tube (Fig. 1-2C). Considered to come from mesenchymal tissue, the notochord stretches from the dorsum sellae in the skull to the coccyx. Around it 30 or more somites form preaxially. In human embryos, the first pair of somites appears at about the 16th day after fertilization.

As the somites mature, a definite cavity, or myocele, appears in the center of each somite. With further growth, the dorsomesial part of the somite forms the skeletal muscles, and it is therefore called the myotome. The ventrolateral portion is called the dermatome or cutis plate. The third region of the somite, the sclerotome, is found ventromesially in a compact mass. These cells become concentrated around the neural tube and notochord and eventually form the vertebrae (Fig. 1-2C).

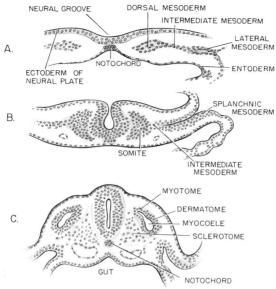

Fig. 1-2. Cross-sectional drawing depicting early development of the notochord, neural groove, somite, and myotome. (From Keim HA: Scoliosis: embryology and anatomy, in The American Academy of Orthopaedic Surgeons: Instructional Course Lectures, vol. XXIV, St. Louis, Mosby, 1975; modified from Patten BM: Human Embryology, Philadelphia, Blakiston, 1952)

The parts of the skeleton that form first are recognizable during the membrane stage, which runs from 21 days to 3 months and is also called the blastemal stage. The part of the sclerotome surrounding the notochord differentiates into the vertebral centrum, which is the body of the vertebra (Fig. 1-3). This condensed mesoderm eventually has two centers of chondrification; the cartilaginous centrum which results then undergoes endochondral ossification from a single ossific center. Between the vertebral centra the sclerotome, as it surrounds the notochord, forms the annulus fibrosus of the intervertebral disc; whereas the notochord in the middle of the disc becomes modified by mucoid degeneration of its cells to form the soft nucleus pulposus. Thus, the notochord persists into adult life not only in this manner, but also as the apical ligament of the odontoid and occasional remnants of the sacrum, skull base, and vertebral bodies.

In Figure 1-3, a longitudinal section through the back of an embryo shows the sclerotomes arranged serially around the length of the notochord. The caudal aspect of each sclerotome becomes condensed by dense cell aggregation. This area becomes demarcated from the cephalic (less condensed) half-

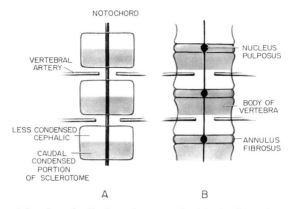

NOTOCHORD

VERTEBRAL
ARTERY

NUCLEUS
PULPOSUS

LESS CONDENSED
CEPHALIC

BODY OF
VERTEBRA

CAUDAL
CONDENSED
PORTION
OF SCLEROTOME

ANNULUS
FIBROSUS

A   B

Fig. 1-3. Longitudinal section; vertebral body formation with entrapment of vertebral artery and formation of nucleus pulposus as notochord remnant. (From Keim HA: Scoliosis: embryology and anatomy, in The American Academy of Orthopaedic Surgeons: Instructional Course Lectures, vol. XXIV, St. Louis, Mosby, 1975; modified from Harrison RG: A Textbook of Human Embryology, Philadelphia, Davis, 1963)

sclerotome. The cephalic part of the caudal condensed portion remains in the middle of the somite and forms the intervertebral disc. The caudal part of the caudal (condensed) half-sclerotome joins with the cephalic (less condensed) portion of the immediately caudal sclerotome to form the vertebral body and traps the intersegmental artery in the center.

The migration of the sclerotome dorsally around the neural tube forms the neural arch of the vertebra; when these paired migrations meet dorsal to the neural tube, they join to form the vertebral spinous process. Failure to meet at the midline leads to spina bifida, in more severe forms, to meningocele. If the neural elements bulge into the meningocele, a myelomeningocele is formed; the resultant neurological deficit is determined by the size of the deformity.

Ossification of the neural arch closely resembles that in the diaphysis of a long bone. Calcification of the cartilaginous matrix is followed by deposition of bone at the surface immediately beneath the periosteum. Therefore, ossification continues by thickening and extension of this subperiosteal bone, while the calcified cartilage enclosed by it is gradually removed. The ossification is not accomplished by two centers of ossification, one for each half of the neural arch, as was formerly thought.

Spinal ossification starts in the midthoracic vertebral bodies at the 8th to 10th week of gestation and gradually involves the vertebra above and below. The ossified marginal ring apophyses begin to fuse with the ossified vertebral body

CONGENITAL SCOLIOSIS

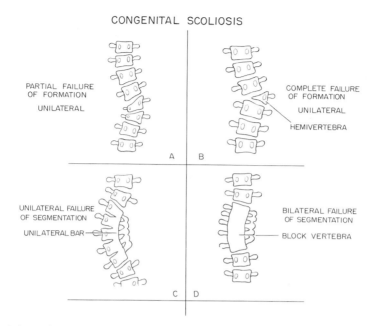

PARTIAL FAILURE
OF FORMATION

UNILATERAL

COMPLETE FAILURE
OF FORMATION

UNILATERAL

HEMIVERTEBRA

A   B

UNILATERAL FAILURE
OF SEGMENTATION

UNILATERAL BAR

BILATERAL FAILURE
OF SEGMENTATION

BLOCK VERTEBRA

C   D

Fig. 1-4. Diagram of failures of formation and segmentation. (From Keim HA: Scoliosis: embryology and anatomy, in The American Academy of Orthopaedic Surgeons: Instructional Course Lectures, vol. XXIV, St. Louis, Mosby, 1975; modified from MacEwen GD.[14])

at the 15th year in girls, a significant time in the pathogenesis of such conditions as scoliosis and kyphosis.

Congenital deformities in the spine can be symptomatic or asymptomatic and can be characterized by fusion, nonfusion, congenital absence, and a myriad of combinations. These anomalies occur when many other important organs and systems are forming. Therefore, a child with spinal anomalies usually has other systemic anomalies, such as cardiac, urinary, or neural problems, which may be asymptomatic but are extremely important clinically. Many anomalous urinary tract problems, such as absent or horseshoe kidneys, have been uncovered during routine intravenous pyelography before surgery in children with congenital spinal problems.

An important aphorism to remember is ''Disorders of migration produce disorders of segmentation.'' This means that congenital spinal disorders can be caused by disturbances of either lateral or longitudinal growth.

Lateral growth anomalies are caused by defects in which the sclerotome fails to migrate across the midline, as in ''wedged'' vertebra (partial unilateral failure of migration and formation; Fig. 1-4A). Also, lateral growth failure can result in hemivertebra (complete unilateral failure of migration and formation; Fig. 1-4B).

Longitudinal growth anomalies can be formed by defects in which the sclerotome fails to segment unilaterally (congenital bar formation; Fig. 1-4C) or in which there is bilateral failure of segmentation ("block" vertebra; Fig. 1-4D).

Often lateral and longitudinal spinal growth is affected, as in common "mixed" vertebral anomalies. These can be extremely complicated with rib fusion and dozens of associated anomalies occurring on both sides of the spine. In some instances, deformed vertebrae can balance each other and result in a straight spine; however, a particularly insidious combination that can cause severe congenital scoliosis is a hemivertebra on one side of the spine and a unilateral bar on the other.

ANATOMY OF THE SPINE

The vertebral column is composed of vertebrae, discs, ligaments, and muscles. Rotation is a normal movement of the thoracic spine. Lateral bending, extension, and forward flexion occur mainly in the lumbar area. Spinal stability is affected by both intrinsic and extrinsic structures, which allow the spine to remain erect and balance the trunk over the pelvis.

Intrinsic stability of the vertebral column is maintained by: (1) the vertebrae and discs—especially the annulus fibrosus; (2) the articular facets of the posterior intervertebral joints and their capsules; (3) the intraspinous and supraspinous ligaments, the ligamenta flava between the laminae, and the posterior and anterior longitudinal ligaments; (4) the small intrinsic intervertebral and erector spinae muscles.

The rib cage provides extrinsic stability of the spine. Each rib is supported by its intercostal muscles and ligaments, which join rib to rib and rib to transverse process and vertebral body. In front, the rib cage is strengthened by the sternum and costal cartilages. The anterior and lateral abdominal muscles also support the spine extrinsically.

The spinal column is a chain of blocks, stacked one on top of the other and kept from collapsing by an exact system of muscles and ligaments that acts with synergistic and antagonistic precision. Thirty-three spinal vertebrae are held together by multiple ligaments and interposed cartilages: seven cervical, twelve thoracic, five lumbar, five sacral (fused into one), and four coccygeal (often fused into one). Since the sacrum and the coccyx are usually each considered as one unit, every human being has, in effect, 26 active vertebrae (Frontispiece).

In the developing fetus, the spinal column forms in the shape of a large kyphotic curve. However, shortly after birth, the spine develops its normal cervical and lumbar lordoses, with compensatory thoracic and sacral kyphoses.

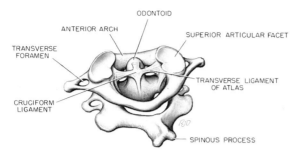

Fig. 1-5. Anatomical alignment of the atlas and axis.

The Cervical Spine

The cervical spine (Figs. 1-5, 1-6) has certain peculiarities at the junction of the head and neck that are essential for proper motion and also for transmission of the neural and vascular elements at the upper part of the spine. The uppermost vertebra, the atlas, has no body and no spinous process but consists mainly of two lateral masses and two arches. The anterior arch of the atlas appears at age 1 and fuses by age 4. The major function at the occiput and atlas is side-to-side rotation of the head. Flexion and extension of the head on the neck are accomplished mainly between the atlas and the axis. The axis is a peculiar vertebra because of the odontoid process that rises perpendicularly from the midportion of the upper surface of its body. In a slight constriction at its base, which is called the neck, is a small groove for the attachment of the transverse atlantal ligament. The odontoid process develops by two bilateral ossification centers, and the line formed by these centers may be present until age 4 or 5. After the age of 7, all epiphyseal centers between the second and seventh cervical vertebrae are usually closed. Generally, by 8 years of age, a child's neck is already in the "adult" form. The spinous process of the axis is usually large, strong, and bifid. Its transverse processes are small but allow

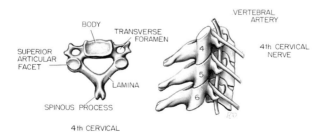

Fig. 1-6. Anatomy of the middle cervical vertebrae (C-4, 5, & 6) with relationship of the vertebral artery to cervical nerves 4, 5, & 6.

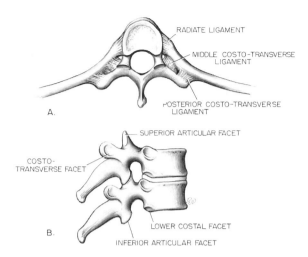

Fig. 1-7. A typical thoracic vertebra showing ligamentous attachment to ribs and articulation with adjoining vertebrae.

room for the vertebral artery to pass through the transverse foramen, which is present in all seven cervical vertebrae. The distinguishing feature of cervical vertebrae three through seven is that the seventh cervical vertebra has a prominent spinous process called the vertebra prominens. The remaining cervical vertebrae have rather common shapes and alignments with smooth bodies that are broader from side to side than in the anteroposterior diameter. The transverse processes in all seven cervical vertebrae contain the vertebral vein and sympathetic nervous pathways. However, the vertebral artery skips the seventh transverse foramen and enters the sixth vertebral foramen as it ascends the cervical spine.

Thoracic Spine

The 12 thoracic vertebrae (Fig. 1-7) are distinctive in that their facets for articulation with the ribs are found on the transverse processes and the vertebral bodies. The upper and lower costal facets, located near the root of the pedicle, serve for articulation with the head of the ribs. The laminae are short and broad and tend to overlap the ones below. The facet joints in the thoracic region overlap each other like shingles on a roof. In contrast, the facet joints in the lower thoracic and lumbar regions are displaced more sagittally and allow for spinal flexion and extension.

The articulation of the ribs to the thoracic vertebrae is of importance in many adolescent pathological conditions. The end of the rib articulates at the junction between two thoracic vertebral bodies. The neck of the rib articulates with the transverse process of the vertebra by a strong ligament network which also holds the rib end to the junction of two vertebral bodies.

Lumbar Spine

The lumbar vertebrae (Fig. 1-8) are large and massive because of their weight-bearing function. They are characterized by the lack of foramina in the transverse processes, such as are found in the cervical spine, and by an absence of articulating facets on the body itself, as are found in the thoracic vertebrae. In the lumbar region, the spinal canal is triangular and smaller than in the cervical spine. The pedicles that arise from the sides of the upper portion of the vertebral body are short and strong, and proceed posteriorly to form the superior and inferior vertebral notches. The inferior portion of the pedicle above and the superior portion of the pedicle below form an intervertebral foramen, through which the spinal nerves exit. In the foramen, the spinal nerves are vulnerable to lesions impinging on the available space, such as tumors, trauma, and degenerative disease. These same processes can also occur in the cervical and thoracic spine.

The facet joints throughout the spine are made up of the inferior facet of the upper vertebra and the superior facet of the lower vertebra. These are true diarthrodial joints, complete with a synovial lining and joint capsule. The joints between two adjacent vertebral bodies are amphiarthrodial joints, much like the symphysis pubis. Within each intervertebral space is an intervertebral disc composed of a central nucleus pulposus (the remnant of the notochord) surrounded by the annulus fibrosus. This fibrocartilaginous disc acts as a shock absorber between adjacent vertebral bodies, and the nucleus pulposus has gelatinous qualities that dissipate mechanical stresses with great efficiency.

A number of important ligaments hold the spinal vertebrae together. The anterior longitudinal ligament runs anterior to the vertebral bodies and is broad and strong, with intimate attachment to each body. The posterior longitudinal ligament is situated along the posterior surface of the vertebral bodies in the anterior surface of the spinal canal. This ligament is considerably weaker than its anterior counterpart. The ligamenta flava, or yellow ligament, connects the laminae of adjacent vertebrae and extends laterally to the articular facets. The supraspinous ligaments join the tips of the spinous processes and are aided in strengthening the spine by the intraspinous ligaments that connect the adjoining spinous processes from their tips to their roots. As mentioned before, the facet joints in the cervical region are arranged in a horizontal or transverse plane, with only a slight posterior-inferior tilt. However, in the thoracic region, the articular facets slope inferiorly like shingles on a roof. In the lumbar region, the articular facets vary considerably from a sagittal disposition at the first and second lumbar vertebrae to an almost coronal position at the lower lumbar

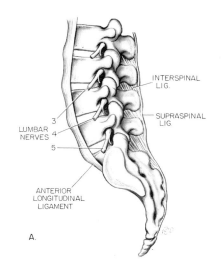

INTERSPINAL
LIG.

SUPRASPINAL
LIG.

3
LUMBAR
NERVES 4

5

ANTERIOR
LONGITUDINAL
LIGAMENT

A.

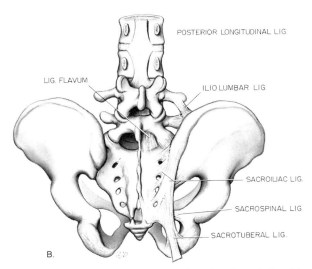

POSTERIOR LONGITUDINAL LIG.

LIG. FLAVUM

ILIO LUMBAR LIG.

SACROILIAC LIG.

SACROSPINAL LIG

SACROTUBERAL LIG.

B.

Fig. 1-8A. Lateral view of lumbar spine showing relationship of
lumbar nerves 3, 4, & 5. B. Posterior view of lower lumbar spine
with articulation to sacrum and pelvis.

10

spine. Sometimes one facet at a specific joint is in the sagittal plane, while the opposite side is in the coronal plane. In the lumbar spine, this is extremely common and is called a facet ''tropism.'' It is suspected to be of clinical significance because it adds rotational stresses to the facet joints.

BLOOD SUPPLY OF THE SPINE

The vascular supply of the vertebral bodies develops through vessels that grow into the ossification centers of the vertebrae. In addition, the vertebral arches have an abundant blood supply. The arteries of the spinal column are segmental from the intercostal arteries, which send a spinal branch through each intervertebral foramen via the posterior branch. Thus, the vertebral bodies are supplied from their outer surfaces, the spinal cord, and the dura.

During embryonic development, blood vessels extend from the outside of the intervertebral disc into the annulus fibrosus but never reach the inner zone, or gelatinous core. These vessels have no connection with the vessels supplying the vertebral bodies. All blood vessels to the discs tend to be obliterated by the 4th year of life. This lack of blood supply to the nucleus pulposus of the intervertebral discs may explain the pathomechanics of disc degeneration in later life, with resultant disc herniation and nerve root compression, which occurs most commonly in the cervical and lumbar spine.

The studies by Adamkiewicz, Kadyi, Bolton, and others form the basis of our knowledge of blood supply to the spinal cord. We have learned mainly that the anterior spinal artery supplies about two-thirds of the cross-sectional area of the spinal cord. Kadyi showed that the anterior spinal artery arises from paired vessels from the vertebral arteries, which pass caudally along the midline of the anterior surface of the spinal cord. Either they unite immediately to form a single vessel, or remain as paired arteries with anastomoses as far as the midcervical region of the cord. This single artery then continues its downward course to be reinforced by feeder vessels in lower areas. Along that course the anterior spinal artery is fed by branches at the level of cervical five or six, and again in the lower thoracic and upper lumbar levels.

The course of the anterior spinal artery in the thoracic region is fairly straight and is as close as possible to the anterior median sulcus. Often a vessel at thoracic four divides into ascending and descending branches of equal diameter—in contrast to the lower thoracic radicular branches, which split into a smaller ascending branch and a larger descending branch. Because the blood supply in the middle thoracic region is so sparse, that area is called the ''watershed'' and is most prone to neurologic damage because of interruption of the blood supply. When vascular interruption destroys the blood supply to the middle thoracic area, the anterior two-thirds of the spinal cord is usually irreversibly damaged.

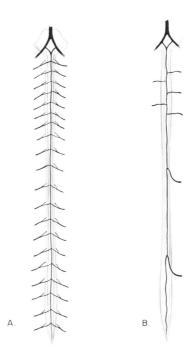

Fig. 1-9A. Original concept of symmetrical segmental blood supply to spinal cord. Each metamere was thought to contribute an individual blood vessel to the spinal cord. *B*. Adamkiewicz proved that only one or two vessels supply the spinal cord in the middle thoracic region. (Reproduced with permission from Doppman, Di Chiro, and Ommaya.[6])

The blood supply to the lower lumbar region is again quite rich, and damage to vessels in that area is not as serious. Therefore, the diameter of the anterior spinal artery varies depending on its proximity to the major arterial feeder. It is largest in the area of the lumbar enlargement and smallest in the midthoracic area of the watershed. The blood flow is downward from the cervical and upper thoracic region and upward from the lumbar region (Fig. 1-9).

According to Gillilan, the ascending course of the artery of Adamkiewicz, which gives it its characteristic hairpin contour, is due to the developmental ascent of the spinal cord. This developmental migration of the cord explains why the cervical contributors of blood supply reach the cord at a horizontal course, while the lower thoracic and lumbar branches must ascend steeply to reach the cord. Injuries to the blood supply of the spinal cord are most common in the midthoracic and lower thoracic regions; this explains why traumatic injury at the level of thoracic twelve or lumbar one often results in paralysis many segments higher than the area of direct trauma.

REFERENCES

1. Adamkiewicz A: Die blutgefasse des menschlicken ruckemarkes. I. Teil. Die gefasse der ruckenmarkssubstanz. Sitzungsb. d.k. Akad. d. Wissensch. Math. Naturw Cl 3 abt Wein 84:496–502, 1882
2. Adamkiewicz A: Die blutgefasse des menschlicken ruckenmarkes. Sitzungsb. d.k. Akad d. Wissensch. Math. Naturw Cl 3 abt Wein 85:101–130, 1882
3. Bolton B: The blood supply of the human spinal cord. J Neurol Neurosurg Psych 2:137–148, 1939
4. Campbell JB: Congenital anomalies of the neural axis. Am J Surg 75:231–256, 1948
5. Cowie TN: Congenital spinal deformities of surgical importance. Acta Radiol 46:38–47, 1956
6. Doppman JL, Di Chiro G, Ommaya AK: Selective Angiography of the Spinal Cord. St. Louis, Green, 1969, pp 3–17
7. Gillilan LA: The arterial blood supply of the human spinal cord. J Comp Neurol 110:75–103, 1958
8. Hamilton WJ, Boyd JD, Mossman HW: Human Embryology, Baltimore, Williams & Wilkins, 1964
9. Horstadius J: The Neural Crest. London, Oxford University Press, 1950
10. James CCM, Lassman LP: Spinal dysraphism. J Bone Joint Surg 44B:208–240, 1962
11. Kadyi H: Uber die Blutgefasse des menschlicken ruckenmarkes. Lemberg, Gubrynowicz and Schmidt, 1889, p 152
12. Keim HA: Scoliosis. Clinical Symposia 24:2–32, CIBA Geigy, 1972
13. Keith A: Human Embryology and Morphology. Baltimore, Williams & Wilkins, 1948
14. MacEwen G Dean: Classification and natural course of congenital scoliosis, in Keim HA (ed): First Annual Postgraduate Course on the Management and Care of the Scoliosis Patient. Warsaw, Indiana, Zimmer, 1969, pp 26–31
15. Patten BM: Foundations of Embryology. New York, McGraw-Hill, 1964
16. Sensenig, EC: Early development of the human vertebral column. Carnegie Inst Contrib Embryol 33:22, 1949

2
Neurology of the Spine

The embryological appearance of a vertebral column marks the beginning of the final stages of neural development. The peripheral nerves develop from cells adjacent to the embryonic neural crest. They develop from ectodermal tissue, continue to proliferate, and eventually lie in long strands along the dorsal aspect of the neural tube. In the developing embryo, nerve elements lie in a homogenous undifferentiated mass at first, but at the limb bud level, sheets of nerve fibers infiltrate the primitive muscle mass around the skeletal core. As the limb grows, the muscle mass develops into individual muscles, drawing the nerve connections with it. The nerve roots around the upper extremities form the brachial plexus, while those around the lower extremities form the lumbosacral plexus.

The formation of the main plexuses can vary because of alterations in the level of limb bud development. Normally, the base of the arm bud is opposite the lower four cervical and first thoracic vertebrae. If this relationship of the vertebral bodies to the axis of the arm varies, nerves from different levels may enter the limb buds. A variation of as many as three segments in the origin of roots entering the limb can occur. When the limb bud is high, a fuller contribution from cervical four enters; consequently, there is less contribution from thoracic one. Such a situation favors a larger rib element at the seventh cervical vertebra because less resistance to the formation of the primitive costal segment is encountered. When this costal element is large, it becomes an obstacle to the plexus, which must then arch up and over the obstruction. This causes a "cervical rib," which results from the so-called "prefixed" plexus (Figs. 2-1, 2-2).

If the limb bud arises at a more caudal level, segments from the lower

15

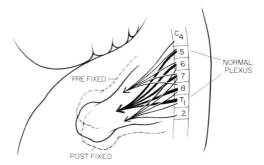

Fig. 2-1. Diagram of normal limb bud with segments coming
from C-5, 6, 7, 8, and T-1. Note also the possibilities of a prefixed
and postfixed brachial plexus. (After Bateman.[1])

spinal cord contribute to the brachial plexus, and the fifth cervical nerve root
and the second thoracic nerve root(s) are most prominent, with little contribution from the fourth cervical segment. This anatomical variation consists of a
"postfixed" plexus, which presents an obstruction to the developing rib elements of the seventh cervical vertebra, and in this case there is no extra cervical
rib. An anatomical fact that is clinically significant is the arrangement of the
cervical nerve roots and the cervical vertebrae. Because there are eight cervical
nerve roots and only seven cervical vertebrae, the first cervical nerve root exits
between the occiput and the atlas, whereas the eighth cervical nerve exits
between the seventh cervical and first thoracic vertebrae (Fig. 2-2). Thus, a
herniated disc at the fifth and sixth cervical vertebrae affects the sixth cervical
nerve as it exits from the spine (Fig. 2-3).

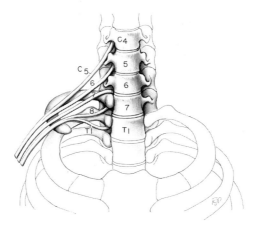

Fig. 2-2. Diagram illustrating relationship of brachial plexus to a
cervical rib.

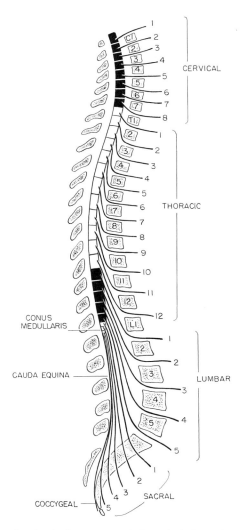

Fig. 2-3. Anatomical arrangement of cervical, thoracic, and lumbar nerves in relation to vertebral bodies. Note that there are 7 cervical vertebrae but 8 cervical nerve roots. Thus, a herniated disc between the bodies of C-5 and C-6 will affect the 6th cervical nerve root. A herniated disc between the bodies of L-4 and 5 will not affect the 4th lumbar nerve root because it has already exited from the spine, but it will affect the 5th lumbar nerve root (see text).

17

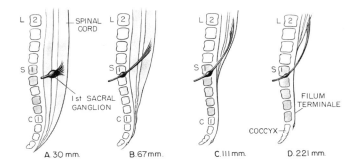

UPWARD MIGRATION OF SPINAL CORD WITH GROWTH

Fig. 2-4. Upward migration of spinal cord with growth. At birth,
spinal cord has migrated to 3rd lumbar vertebra; by age 5 it is
usually at the level of 2nd lumbar vertebra; by adulthood, it has
ascended between L-1 and L-2. (From Keim HA: Scoliosis: embryology and anatomy, in The American Academy of Orthopaedic
Surgeons: Instructional Course Lectures, vol. XXIV, St. Louis,
Mosby, 1975; modified from Patten BM: Human Embryology.
Philadelphia, Blakiston, 1952)

The first thoracic nerve exits through the intervertebral foramen, made up
of the first and second thoracic vertebrae, and the twelfth thoracic nerve exits
between the twelfth thoracic and the first lumbar vertebrae.

However, in the lumbar region the anatomy changes drastically. Although
the fourth lumbar nerve root does emerge from the foramen formed by the
pedicles of the fourth and fifth lumbar vertebrae, it is not the nerve root usually
affected by a herniation of the fourth lumbar disc. A disc herniation at this level
actually affects the fifth lumbar nerve root because of the continuing upward
migration of the conus medullaris from fetal life to maturity. Because skeletal
growth is greater than neural growth, the conus medullaris migrates from the tip
of the coccyx in the fetus at 3 months to the upper border of the third lumbar
vertebra at birth. By the time a child is 5 years old, the lower tip of the spinal
cord is usually at the level of the second lumbar vertebra, and by adulthood, the
conus is at the lower border of the first lumbar vertebra (Fig. 2-4).

This upward cord migration during development causes the lumbar nerve
roots to slant downward at an acute angle. Thus, a disc herniation between the
fourth and fifth lumbar vertebrae does not affect the fourth lumbar nerve root
(which has already exited), but usually causes pressure on the fifth lumbar
nerve root on its way caudally to exit between the fifth lumbar vertebra and the
sacrum. Likewise, a disc herniation between the fifth lumbar vertebra and the
sacrum usually affects the first sacral nerve root and not the fifth lumbar nerve
root, as might be expected.

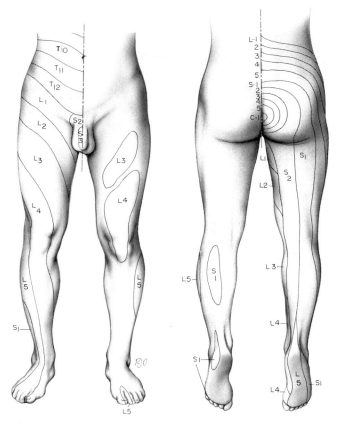

Fig. 2-5.   The sensory dermatomes. (Modified after Keegan and
Garrett.[3])

The neurological application of anatomical facts can be most helpful when
clinically applied. A deficit of most spinal nerves can be readily localized
through a good sensory examination (Fig. 2-5). This can also be said for an
orderly sequence in the motor innervation of the limb musculature.

Unfortunately, physicians have always had to memorize long tables of
nerve innervation into muscles, as well as the muscular distribution of each
spinal root or limb plexus, which is difficult and meaningless. Because there is
lack of correspondence between overlying dermatomes and underlying
myotomes, the orderly arrangement of dermatomes seems to cover a bewilder-
ing and chaotic distribution of myotomes.

However, if the fundamental manner in which joint movements are
segmentally innervated is appreciated, the complex subject of muscle innervation becomes rational and can be mastered quickly.

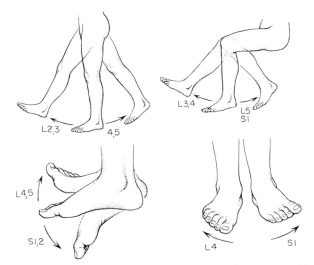

Fig. 2-6. Diagram of segmental innervation to lower extremities (see text). (Modified after Last.[5])

Generally, any movement of a joint is innervated by two adjoining segments (although this is less true in the upper extremities). The four segments activated in a movement and its opposite are in numerical sequence and control all possible movements in the joint (Fig. 2-6). For example, the spinal center of the hip joint includes lumbar segments two, three, four, and five, of which lumbar segments two and three control flexion, medial rotation, and adduction, while lumbar segments four and five control the opposite movements—extension, lateral rotation, and abduction.

Also, in passing distally by one joint into a limb, the four segments comprising joint innervation are one segment lower in the spinal cord. Thus, the center for the knee is lumbar three, four, and five, and sacral nerve root one. It also follows that the ankle joint, which is one joint lower in the limb, has a center one segment lower—namely, lumbar four and five and sacral nerve roots one and two. Thus, four spinal segments control the hip, knee, and ankle: the hip is innervated by lumbar two, three, four, and five; the knee by lumbar three, four, five, and sacral one; the ankle by lumbar four and five and sacral one and two.

Therefore, knowledge of the primary action of any muscle is all that is required to determine its nerve supply. For example, the psoas and iliacus muscles flex the hip and therefore are supplied by the second and third lumbar nerve roots. The vastus intermedius extends the knee and is thus innervated by the third and fourth lumbar nerve roots. The soleus muscle plantar flexes the ankle, so it receives its neural stimulation from the first and second sacral

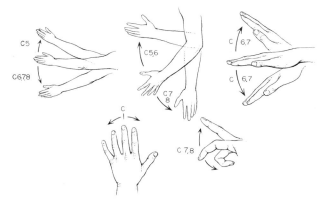

Fig. 2-7. Diagram of segmental innervation to the upper extremities. (See text.) (Modified after Last.[5])

nerves. Finally, the extensor hallucis longus extends the great toe and is innervated solely by the fifth lumbar nerve. In patients with a herniated disc between the fourth and fifth lumbar vertebrae, the fifth lumbar nerve root is involved, and the extensor hallucis longus is weakened. The concurrent sensory deficit in such patients is in a small autonomous zone of the fifth lumbar nerve at the web space between the great and second toes.

In the upper extremities, the rule that each joint movement is controlled through two contiguous spinal segments does not hold as universally as in the lower extremities. In most cases, the essential segment is a single one, but joints further down the limb generally are controlled by spinal centers lower in the cord. The segments controlling the joints of the upper limb are shown in their simplest form in Figure 2-7. Thus, the shoulder abducts and externally rotates with cervical nerve root five; whereas it adducts and internally rotates with roots six, seven, and eight. The elbow, which is one joint lower, flexes due to nerve roots five and six, and extends due to nerve roots seven and eight. The forearm pronates and supinates with cervical nerve root six. The wrist flexes and extends with cervical nerve roots six and seven, with the fingers flexing and extending with cervical nerves seven and eight. The intrinsic muscles of the hand basically are innervated by the first thoracic nerve.

Although it may be objected that the deltoid receives segments from cervical five and six, and not merely cervical five, we know anatomically that muscles may receive fibers from several nerve roots, but usually all of these roots are not equally significant. The most significant innervation of the deltoid muscle is cervical root five. The constitution of the phrenic nerve illustrates this point. The phrenic nerve is composed of elements from cervical nerve roots three, four, and five. However, the most essential segment is from cervical nerve four, for without it the diaphragm cannot function. The outlying scheme illustrated here is intended to indicate the most essential segments of innervation with sufficient accuracy for clinical purposes. For the clinician and student, this scheme provides a simple way to remember the segmental supply of any limb muscle and the muscular distribution of any spinal segment.

A complete physical examination of any adolescent patient includes a thorough neurological evaluation. After he has gathered a thorough history, including the chief complaint, the physician should also evaluate the past history, with special emphasis on previous trauma, illness, or surgical procedures. Next, a good examination should be performed, which includes muscle testing for motor power, sensory evaluation, and, finally, evaluation of all major reflexes in the upper and lower extremities. A Romberg test should always be performed.

A good clinical understanding of the segmental innervation of the muscles in the upper and lower extremities can make the clinical examination of the patient easier and more pleasurable.

REFERENCES

1. Bateman JE: Trauma to Nerves in Limbs. Philadelphia, Saunders, 1962, pp 3–12
2. Ford FR: Diseases of the Nervous System in Infancy, Childhood and Adolescence. Springfield, Illinois, Thomas, 1961
3. Keegan J, Garrett F: The segmental distribution of the cutaneous nerves in the limbs of man. Anat Rec 102:409, 1948
4. Keim HA: Low back pain. Clinical Symposia 25,3:2–8, CIBA Geigy, 1973
5. Last RJ: Innervation of the limbs. J Bone Joint Surg 31B:452–464, 1949
6. Manter JT, Gatz AJ: Clinical Neuroanatomy and Neurophysiology, ed 2. Philadelphia, Davis, 1964, pp 1–35
7. Netter FH: Nervous System. The CIBA Collection of Medical Illustrations. New York, Colorpress, 1957, pp 49–55
8. Wells JL: Development of the human diaphragm. Carnegie Inst Contrib Embryol 35:107, 1954

3
The So-Called Normal Adolescent Spine

POSTURE

Before designating certain posture as good or bad, one must define the term posture. Without considering physiologic correctness, we must first define posture as the expression of the body's equilibrium and balance. In contrast, locomotion expresses a rhythmic play between the loss and recovery of balance. In static posture, the individual is at rest and his balance is secure. During locomotion, the individual's balance is overthrown by the moving body, which constantly attempts to reinstate balance.

Normal human posture is the end result of generations of transformation from the quadruped to the bipedalistic balance of man. To consider posture as a thoroughly stable anatomical fact would be to misunderstand its evolutionary character. Therefore, normal posture is a physiologic state with some latitude, and we should not think of it as a fixed or rigid condition. It is better to speak of a normal range of posture—that is, a field of individual variation within which posture may swing back and forth and still be within the framework of what we call normal.

Three main areas determine man's ability to walk and stand upright: strong extensors around the hip; the extensors of the spine; and the inclination of the pelvis (normally about 60° to the horizontal plane when the body is upright).

The center of gravity normally extends from the mastoid process of the skull slightly posterior to the cervical spine, then slightly anterior to the thoracic spine. It bisects the thoracolumbar junction and runs between the sacroiliac axis and just posterior to the center of the hip joint. The axis then continues

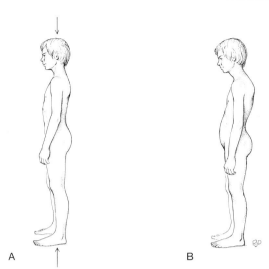

Fig. 3-1A.   Normal posture in the adolescent. Note proper relationship of center of gravity to various anatomical portions of spine
and pelvis. B. Abnormal posture in the adolescent, showing marked
increase of thoracic kyphosis and lumbar lordosis.

downward immediately in front of the knee joint axis and passes through the
front of the talus between the feet. This condition is referred to as normal
distribution of gravitational forces (Fig. 3-1A). The weight-bearing center of
the body is just in front of the fourth lumbar vertebra. Even a considerable
degree of lumbar lordosis can be compensated for by an increase of the normal
thoracic kyphosis to keep the center of gravity in the same position.

Although specific pathologic postural types were described by Lovett,
Willis, and Steindler, the most common cause of mechanical back pain in the
adult occurs from poor posture habits learned in childhood and adolescence.
This posture is best shown in Figure 3-1B and consists of increased anterior
inclination of the head, increased cervical lordosis, and thoracic kyphosis. The
chest is sunken, the abdomen protrudes, and as adults gain weight through
aging and lack of regular daily exercise, lumbar lordosis increases. The
resulting swayback and protruding buttock are necessary and compensatory to
balance the center of gravity and contribute to more anatomical sag and
weakness in the supporting muscles of the trunk and pelvis.

Poor posture often starts in early childhood and causes great friction
between parents and child. While on the telephone or watching television,
children can assume postural configurations that would confound the most
supple guru. To slouch in a chair or school seat is the ''accepted'' way to sit,
and children who are not athletically inclined are especially prone to develop
posture that plagues them throughout their adult life.

Family physicians and pediatricians must be especially aware of good posture and insist that parents enforce correct attitudes in rearing their children. Numerous corrective exercises and techniques are available to teach proper body grace and posture. These are effective and can be used along with dance classes and athletics to help the growing body develop into a model for adult growth and normal, painless function. Children rarely complain of backache from poor posture. In adults, however, poor posture is frequently the cause of low back strain and pain.

Treatment of poor posture includes passive and active exercises. Any contracted soft tissues—such as hamstrings, hip flexors, lumbosacral fascia, pectorals, or neck flexors—should be stretched passively. The patient is instructed to perform daily exercises to increase motor strength of key muscles affecting posture, especially the abdominal muscles (sit-ups, kicking, and bicycling), gluteus maximus (hip extension against gravity with knees in flexion), erector spinae (hyperextension of the spine against gravity in the prone position), and scapular adductors (bring shoulder blades backward toward the midline in the prone or sitting position).

The most important exercise to correct lumbar lordosis is the pelvic tilt, in which the patient decreases pelvic inclination by using the abdominal and gluteus maximus muscles. Initially, the pelvic tilt exercises are performed in the supine position, then finally standing against the wall. By reducing the pelvic tilt, the patient decreases all exaggerated curves of the spine. The shoulders are brought over the pelvis with the head held erect and the chin in. These exercises are performed daily until the patient can maintain correct posture naturally and develop a normal stance and gait.

REFERENCES

1. Krusen FH, Kottke FJ, Ellwood PM: Handbook of Physical Medicine and Rehabilitation. Philadelphia, Saunders, 1965, pp 607–613
2. Lovett RW: Lateral Curvature of the Spine and Round Shoulders. New York, Blakiston, 1916
3. Steindler A: Diseases and Deformities of the Spine and Thorax. St. Louis, Mosby, 1929, pp 87–125
4. Steindler A: Kinesiology of the Human Body. Springfield, Illinois, Thomas, 1955
5. Taylor HL: Standardization of conditions affecting posture. J Orth Surg 14:569, 1916

4

Congenital Problems in the Adolescent Spine

Congenital abnormalities are defects in the development of body form or function that are present at birth. The embryological development of the spinal column is complex, as was mentioned in the section on embryology, and is closely related to the development of the spinal cord, heart, great vessels, and genitourinary system, which lie adjacent to the spinal column. Developmental anomalies in the spinal column are frequently associated with central nervous system malformations and abnormalities of cardiac and renal development. Only certain congenital conditions are mentioned in this chapter, and those related to scoliosis and kyphosis are described in subsequent chapters.

KLIPPEL-FEIL SYNDROME

The Klippel-Feil syndrome (also known as congenital synostosis of the cervical vertebrae, or brevicollis) is a rare malformation in which there is a congenital fusion of two or more vertebrae in the cervical region. The syndrome is manifested clinically by shortening of the neck and limitation of its motion. The first complete clinical description of this syndrome was given by Klippel and Feil in 1912. The patient was a 46-year-old tailor who appeared to have a short neck, restricted head movement, and a hairline extending to the thorax. Dissection revealed four cervical vertebrae, each with bilateral cervical ribs and spina bifida occulta that was called a ''cervical thorax'' (Fig. 4-1 A,B).

The Klippel-Feil syndrome results from a failure of normal segmentation of the mesodermal somites during the 3rd to the 8th weeks of fetal life, the exact

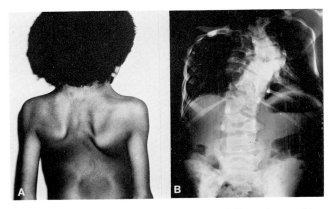

Fig. 4-1*A*. 11-year old boy with Klippel-Feil syndrome. Note elevation of left scapula (Sprengel's deformity). *B*. X-ray of same patient showing multiple severe congenital anomalies: many hemivertebrae, block vertebrae, and unilateral bars throughout thoracic and lumbar spine. Note congenital fusion of transverse processes of lower lumbar vertebrae.

cause of which is still subject to conjecture. No definite pattern of inheritance has been established; however, several instances of Klippel-Feil syndrome in the same family have been recorded. The condition is more prominent in women.

In more involved cases, the neck is short and the head appears to sit directly on the thorax. There is marked limitation of motion of the cervical spine, with flexion and extension taking place mostly between the occiput and atlas. The webbing of the soft tissues on each side of the neck extends from the mastoid processes to the acromion of the shoulders and is sometimes referred to as pterygium colli.

Hensinger, Lang, and MacEwen recently studied 50 patients with this syndrome. They concluded that the cervical lesion and the attendant clinical findings are relatively minor disabilities compared to associated anomalies in other areas. These include a 60 percent incidence of scoliosis, of which half of the patients required bracing or surgery; 35 percent had abnormalities of the urinary tract, and 30 percent had a hearing impairment; 18 percent exhibited "mirror motions" (synkinesia) of the upper extremities, 14 percent had congenital cardiovascular disease, and 40 percent had Sprengel's deformity (congenital elevation of the scapula).

In mild cases, treatment consists of passive stretching exercises to obtain the maximum range of motion. Surgery is almost always needed in advanced cases, especially in forms of torticollis. Corrective surgery can be maintained by use of a Milwaukee brace postoperatively, especially since these patients often also have scoliosis and kyphosis.

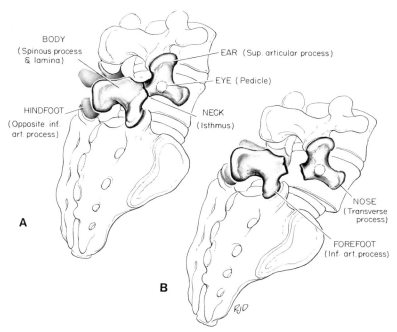

Fig. 4-2. Spondylolysis and spondylolisthesis showing typical ''Scottie dog'' profile of posterior elements of 5th lumbar vertebra, seen on an oblique x-ray view. A collar is around Scottie dog's neck in spondylolysis; complete amputation of dog's neck indicates spondylolisthesis.

Surgical efforts are usually directed toward improving appearance and function, with Z-plasty of muscle and fascial areas to allow greater freedom of neck movement. Cervical ribs, which are sometimes associated, are described in the section on neurology (Chapter 2). If these ribs cause brachial plexus problems, they can also be resected.

SPONDYLOLISTHESIS

Historically, the term spondylolisthesis is derived from the Greek word *spondylos*, meaning ''spine,'' and *olisthanein*, meaning ''to slip.'' The condition was originally noted by obstetricians, but Andre described a condition called ''hollow back'' as early as 1741 and defined it as inward warping of the spine. In 1855 Robert was the first to focus attention on the lesion in the neural arch and carefully dissected the 5th lumbar vertebra to demonstrate that a vertebrae with an intact neural arch could not slip forward. The discontinuity in the pars interarticularis was demonstrated by Lambl in 1858 (Fig. 4-2).

In 1834 Kilian coined the term spondylolisthesis for a forward slip of one vertebra on another. This condition should not be confused with spondylolysis, which is merely a defect in the pars interarticularis, or isthmus, of a vertebra. In spondylolysis there is no forward slipping, and this condition does not necessarily proceed to spondylolisthesis. The most common location for spondylolisthesis is between lumbar five and the sacrum, followed by lumbar four on five; however, the condition has been described even in the cervical spine.

Newman and Stone's description of the five types of spondylolisthesis has helped elucidate the cause of this condition and has contributed to proper treatment and management. In Newman's type one, "congenital" spondylolisthesis, the slipping occurs at the lumbosacral junction and is due to a congenital sacral defect, including the articular facets with attenuation of the neural arch. The arch is rarely broken but appears "stretched out" and elongated (Fig. 4-3 B).

Type two, or "spondylolytic," spondylolisthesis, is "true" spondylolisthesis, with slipping of the vertebrae due to a break of the pars interarticularis (Fig. 4-3 C). Many authorities consider the break to be a stress fracture. Type two is most common in Caucasian men and least common in Negro women. The facets remain intact, and the degree of slip is classified from grades I through IV, with grade I being a slip of 25 percent of the vertebral body below, and grade IV slip being a complete slip with the superior vertebral body directly anterior to the vertebral body or sacrum below it. (Fig. 4-4).

Type three, "traumatic" spondylolisthesis, is slipping due to instability caused by an acute fracture of the neural arch and is sometimes seen in seatbelt injuries in high-speed automobile accidents (Fig. 4-3 D). Type four, "degenerative" spondylolisthesis, is also known as pseudospondylolisthesis, described by Junghanns in 1931, and spondylolisthesis with an intact neural arch, described by Macnab in 1950. Slipping is due to facet deficiency caused by degenerative joint changes and almost always occurs at the fourth lumbar level. Type four is nine times more common in women than in men; it is rarely encountered in the adolescent spine and is usually seen in patients over 40 (Fig. 4-3 E).

Type five, "pathologic" spondylolisthesis, is rare and is characterized by forward slipping due to insufficiency of posterior bony elements that have been eroded by the pathologic process. These also are rarely seen in the adolescent, since bone tumors in that region are rare in adolescents. However, pathologic spondylolisthesis is seen in osteogenesis imperfecta and tuberculosis (Fig. 4-3 F).

Patients with spondylolisthesis often complain of back pain and hamstring muscle spasms. The adolescent usually cannot bend forward with the knees straight and has a stiff spine on examination. If the patient is allowed to bend his knees, the spine can be bent forward, since bending the knees releases the

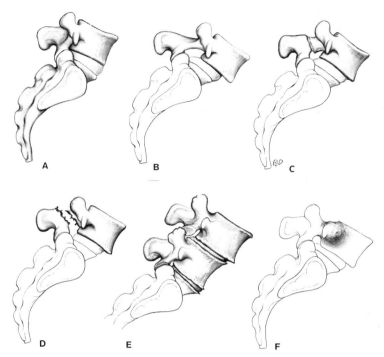

Fig. 4-3.   Newman's 5 types of spondylolisthesis. *A*. Normal relationship. *B*. In type one (congenital), attenuated pars interarticularis stretches into a long, thin structure but usually remains intact. *C*. Type two, spondylolytic spondylolisthesis, or true spondylolisthesis. A break in pars interarticularis (isthmus) allows vertebral body to slide forward, while most posterior elements remain intact. *D*. Type three, traumatic spondylolisthesis, usually occurs with an avulsion type fracture through pars interarticularis. *E*. Type four, degenerative spondylolisthesis. Degenerative changes in facet joints cause joint deficiency or laxity. *F*. Type five, pathologic spondylolisthesis. Forward slipping is due to a defect in vertebral pedicle. Neoplasm or developmental defect allows body of affected vertebra to slide forward. (Redrawn from Newman.[23])

hamstrings. Many adolescents with spondylolisthesis are asymptomatic, and the lesion is detected only in conjunction with other x-rays, such as in a scoliosis examination. (The incidence of spondylolisthesis in scoliosis is 5 percent.) All examinations of the thoracic or lumbar spine should include a spot lateral x-ray of the lumbosacral junction. However, a physician with a keen eye can sometimes diagnose spondylolisthesis on an "A-P" x-ray because of the appearance of the inverted Napoleon hat sign, which is seen in more advanced grades of slippage (Fig. 4-5). This sign is present because the body of the slipped vertebra is superimposed on the vertebra below it and gives the charac-

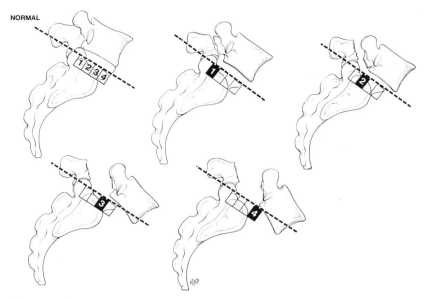

NORMAL

Fig. 4-4. Classification of spondylolisthesis. Grade I, anterior displacement of 25% of vertebral body on one below it. Grade II, displacement of 25–50% of vertebra below. Grade III, 50–75% displacement. Grade IV, greater than 75% displacement, and vertebral body may lie in front of vertebra below. (Redrawn after Meyerding HW: Spondylolisthesis. Surg Gynecol Obstet 54:371, 1932.)

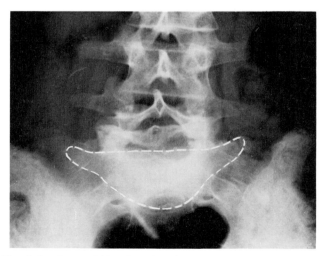

Fig. 4-5. Inverted Napoleon hat sign of spondylolisthesis. Body of lumbar 5 has slid anterior to sacrum, giving superimposed image of hat worn during Napoleon's time. This sign is generally seen only in grades III and IV.

teristic "Napoleon hat" appearance. The best views to represent spondylolis-thesis accurately are right and left oblique x-rays of the area.

In spondylolytic spondylolisthesis (Newman's type two), the defect is usually not present at birth and seldom appears before the age of 4 years. Between the ages of 5½ and 6½, the incidence rises precipitously. Slipping occurs generally before the age of 20, and the period of most rapid slip is between the ages of 10 and 15. The slipping rarely increases after the age of 20.

After extensively studying the etiology of spondylolytic spondylolis-thesis, Wiltse formulated the theory that the defect in the pars interarticularis is caused by two factors: an inherited dysplasia or defect in the cartilage model of the arch of the affected vertebrae, and a fatigue or stress fracture of the weakened pars interarticularis from physical forces resulting from man's characteristic stance and erect posture. Wiltse feels that stress and strain on the pars interarticularis do not produce a defect unless a dysplasia or hereditary weakness is already present. The incidence of this type of spondylolisthesis is higher in adolescent football players—especially in the linemen who subject their spines to shearing stresses during blocking and tackling.

Treatment

An adolescent with painful spondylolisthesis can be watched with serial x-rays at 6-month intervals. If the forward slip increases from grade I onward, the patient should have a posterior fusion to the sacrum to stabilize the slipped fifth lumbar vertebra. The author prefers a fusion from lumbar four to the sacrum since the transverse processes of lumbar four are more accessible than those of lumbar five, and because the fusion prevents disc degeneration at the lumbar four-five level.

If there are no nerve root symptoms, nerve root decompression and removal of the loose posterior elements of the affected vertebra are not per-formed. A bilateral-lateral transverse process fusion is performed using au-togenous iliac crest bone. When there are radicular root symptoms, the loose posterior elements are completely removed and a bilateral foramenotomy is performed to free the impinged nerve roots. The spine is then fused in the bilateral-lateral manner to the sacrum, leaving the midline open and free of bony fragments (Fig. 4-6 A, B, C).

Often the posterior elements of the spine are so loose that they rock back and forth, causing a fibrocartilaginous mass to form at the junction of the posterior vertebral arch and the pars interarticularis. This fibrocartilaginous material usually causes impingement of the nerve roots. When the material is cleared away and a foramenotomy performed, the patient's symptoms usually disappear.

Postoperatively, the patients do not need casts or braces and are encour-aged to start muscle-strengthening exercises. However, for grade III or IV slips

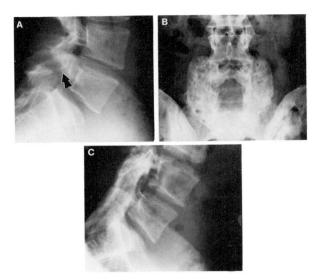

Fig. 4-6A.   Spondylolytic (''isthmic'') spondylolisthesis with defect in pars interarticularis of lumbar 5; grade I slip. *B*. A-P x-ray
showing bilateral-lateral fusion of lumbar 4 to sacrum. Posterior
elements of lumbar 5 were removed and nerve roots cleared by
foramenotomy on both sides. *C*. Lateral view, note new bone added
posteriorly to keep lumbar 5 from sliding further forward.

a plaster cast extending from the nipple line down one thigh to above the knee is
used, and the patient ambulates in this position for 6 months. In unstable grade
IV slips, a 3- to 4-month recumbency period is sometimes necessary to prevent
further slipping during the healing phase of the spinal fusion (Fig. 4-7 A, B, C).

TRANSITIONAL VERTEBRAE

Variations in developmental cogenital defects are seen in many patients
with painful symptoms in the lower spine. Facet tropisms allow one facet joint
in the lumbar vertebrae to be in the sagittal plane, while the other facet joint can
be in the coronal plane. This extremely common tropism is suspected to be of
clinical significance because it adds torque and rotational stress to the facet
joints. However, another condition, sacralization of the fifth lumbar vertebra,
can occur unilaterally or bilaterally. The unilateral condition can be only partial
and allows for formation of a diarthrodial joint in connection with the lateral
mass of the sacrum. Pain generally accompanies the condition, and the
hemisacralization can cause pain down the first sacral nerve root. The condition
is particularly painful when the fifth lumbar transverse process partially articu-

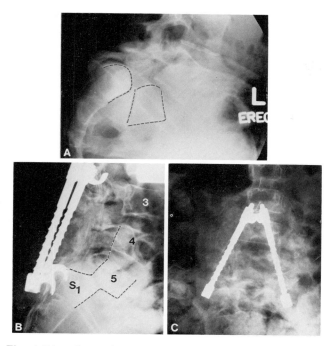

Fig. 4-7A.   Congenital spondylolisthesis; grade IV slip. Note long, stretched out pars interarticularis of lumbar 5, which remains intact. Superior surface of sacrum is rounded. Body of lumbar 5 is trapezoid and anterior to sacrum. B. Lateral x-ray after surgical fusion using 2 Harrington rods to reduce the slip. C. Postoperative A-P view showing Harrington rods in position with bilateral-lateral fusion from lumbar 3 to sacrum.

lates on one side and is free on the other. A powerful leverage is therefore produced on side-bending, with the articulating side acting as a fulcrum (Fig. 4-8).

A syndrome of neuralgic symptoms called Bertolotti's syndrome is considered to be the effect of such a sacralization. The "syndrome" consists of sciatic pain down the leg opposite the sacralized side. Casolo found sacralization in the x-rays of 2.5 percent of a great number of patients screened, with symmetrical sacralization much more common than asymmetrical or unilateral sacralization. Accordingly, 58 percent of those individuals showed x-ray evidence of sacralization and had neurologic symptoms in the form of Bertolotti's syndrome. When both transverse processes of lumbar five are fused to the sacrum, the condition is called total sacralization and usually is not associated with lumbar pain. In these cases, only four lumbar vertebrae are counted. It is also possible to have six lumbar vertebrae and only four sacral

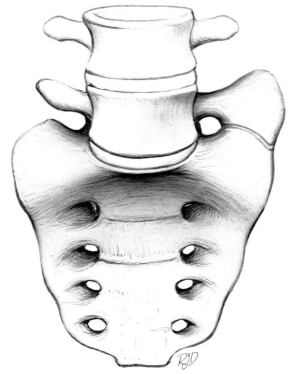

Fig. 4-8.   Unilateral sacralization of transverse process of lumbar
5 to sacrum.

vertebrae (fused into one). If all six vertebrae move and articulate freely, no
pain should occur. However, people with a longer lumbar "lever arm" (six
lumbar vertebrae) are more prone to develop low back pain in later life because
of increased leverage on the lumbar vertebrae and facet joints.

A "sacralized" vertebra usually does not cause pain in itself; however, it
causes abnormal torque to be transmitted to the vertebra above it, and when
associated with a herniated disc, the protrusion is usually on the side opposite
the sacralization and a level above it.

SPINAL DYSRAPHISM

The term spinal dysraphism has been used loosely to include many types
of spinal disorders that can lead to difficulties in and around the spine and lower
extremities. It generally includes all forms of spina bifida, meningocele,
myelomeningocele, and diastematomyelia. Other rare conditions can also be

included under this general heading, but only these main forms will be discussed. Since most of these conditions are well controlled by adolescence, the details of the neonate and infant will not be described.

Spina Bifida

Spina bifida is the most common congenital abnormality of the spine and includes varying degrees of incomplete bony closure of one or more neural arches. The defect can occur at any level, but the most frequent site is in the lumbosacral region, which is usually the last part of the vertebral column to close. Spina bifida occulta is extremely common, but spina bifida with obvious defects is said to have an incidence of 2 out of every 1000 births.

The most important aspect of spina bifida is not the bony loss or instability but the frequently associated neurologic deficit, which is due to incomplete development of the spinal cord (myelodysplasia). When myelodysplasia occurs in forms of meningocele or myelomeningocele, the neurological deficit may vary from mild muscular imbalance and sensory loss in the lower limbs to complete paraplegia, usually at the level of the lesion. Consequently, when spinal deformities or defects in the lower extremities are noted, the spine should be thoroughly examined to rule out an obscure diagnostic problem with neurological sequelae. Bladder and bowel incontinence usually indicates a defect in the lower spinal region. In short, when a patient with a foot deformity is seen, always do a neurological examination and take an x-ray of the spine.

Spina Bifida Occulta

Spina bifida occulta is the mildest degree of spina bifida, which occurs without any external manifestation and is truly undetectable except by x-ray examination (Fig. 4-9). This common form of spina bifida occurs in about 10 percent of the population and is generally not serious, since it is rarely associated with any type of nerve damage or deficit. However, spina bifida occulta is 13 times more frequent with defects of the pars interarticularis and may have some connection with spondylolisthesis.

As mentioned in the chapter on anatomy and embryology, most forms of spinal dysraphism can be explained by an aberration in embryological development—a persistent neurenteric canal—which transiently connects the yolk sac (the future intestinal cavity) through the primitive knot (Hensen's node) to the amnion. The primitive knot migrates distally and ultimately comes to lie in the region of the coccyx before it disappears.

If a neurenteric canal were to arise during development at any location along the spine, and if it were not completely obliterated, it could cause many anomalies of the cord and spine in the form of neural and bone defects and

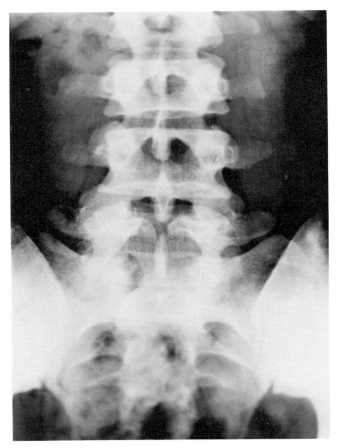

Fig. 4-9.   Spina bifida occulta of lumbar 5. Note defect where posterior elements of 5th lumbar vertebra failed to join in midline during embryonic development.

fistulous connections (Fig. 4-10). These conditions include spina bifida, myelomeningocele, butterfly vertebra, hemivertebra, failure of vertebral segmentation, prevertebral and postvertebral cysts, and diastasis of the spinal cord, as well as diastematomyelia.

Spina Bifida with Meningocele

In spina bifida with meningocele, the meninges extrude through a defect in the neural arches, thereby forming a meningocele covered by normal skin and containing cerebrospinal fluid and some nerve roots. The spinal cord remains

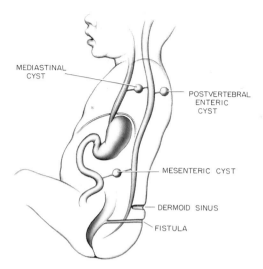

MEDIASTINAL
CYST

POSTVERTEBRAL
ENTERIC
CYST

MESENTERIC CYST

DERMOID SINUS

FISTULA

Fig. 4-10. Sagittal drawing showing multiple cystic anomalies that develop because of persistent connection between neural and enteric canals. Fistulas fail to close during embryonic development, leading to many possible conditions such as mediastinal cysts, diastematomyelia, and dermoid sinuses. (From Keim HA: Scoliosis: embryology and anatomy, In The American Academy of Orthopaedic Surgeons: Instructional Course Lectures, vol. XXIV, St. Louis, Mosby, 1975.)

confined to the spinal canal, and usually little neurologic deficit is detectable at birth. Some types of external skin manifestations commonly noted are lipomas, hemangiomas, dermoid cysts, and hair growth on the external skin.

Spina Bifida with Myelomeningocele

When the abnormality is more severe, the spinal cord and nerve roots are involved and can lie completely within the sac that protrudes from the spine or can be part of the wall of the sac. The overlying membranous sac is sometimes extremely thin and ulcerates easily. In severe myelomeningocele, the skin may be absent, in which case the cord is covered by the arachnoid and is open to serious infections.

Almost all grades of myelomeningocele are accompanied by severe and progressive nerve root involvement. The paralysis is usually flaccid, whereas in spinal cord involvement paralysis is usually of a spastic type. Thus, any child can have both flaccid and spastic paralysis (Fig. 4-11 A, B). Most children with myelomeningocele develop hydrocephalus, which is usually secondary to downward prolongation of the brain stem and part of the cerebellum through the

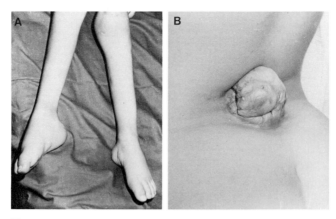

Fig. 4-11.   Child with severe myelomeningocele showing thinned
skin in lower lumbar region. Spinal elements are absent in this area
and have led to almost total paralysis in the lower extremities. Note
atrophy of calves and feet.

foramen magnum. If hydrocephalus progresses because of continued growth of
the spinal vertebral elements and tethering of the spinal cord, an Arnold-Chiari
malformation (descent of the brain stem through the foramen magnum) can
develop, leading to death.

Many operative procedures have been devised in recent years to allow
shunting of the cerebrospinal fluid to the retroperitoneal or venous system, and
many children who normally would have died with myelomeningocele and
severe neurologic and cephalic deficits are now living into adolescent life.
Figure 4-12 shows the effects of nerve root involvement in these conditions.

In almost all forms of myelomeningocele, the neurologic deficit leads to
dislocation of the hips as well as to many other lower-extremity deficiencies.
The patients almost always develop spinal problems that persist into adolescence and early adult life, and they usually develop rather severe forms of
scoliosis. The team approach is important in treating these patients since most
patients have bladder paralysis and need urinary diversion procedures because
of incontinence. If a team is composed of orthopedist, neurosurgeon, urologist,
physiatrist, orthotist, physiotherapist, and cooperative nurses, the patient can
often achieve a fairly normal adolescent and adult life. Through a combination
of surgery, bracing, and enormous attention to physical therapeutics, most
patients can lead reasonably functional lives, but the road is long and difficult.

Diastematomyelia

Diastematomyelia is an uncommon congenital anomaly of the spinal cord.
It has been described by Neuhauser and associates as a congenital malformation
of the neural axis characterized by a sagittal division of a segment of the spinal

Neuro-Segmental Level	HIP	KNEE	ANKLE	FOOT	TOES
L-1	WEAK FLEXION (ILIOPSOAS)				
L-2	FLEXION (ILIOPSOAS AND SARTORIUS) ADDUCTION (ADDUCTOR MUSCLES)	WEAK EXTENSION (QUADRICEPS FEMORIS)			
L-3	FLEXION (ILIOPSOAS AND SARTORIUS) ADDUCTION (ADDUCTOR MUSCLES)	EXTENSION (QUADRICEPS FEMORIS)			
L-4	ABDUCTION (TENSOR FASCIAE LATAE AND GLUTEUS MEDIUS AND MAXIMUS)	STRONG EXTENSION (QUADRICEPS FEMORIS)	DORSI-FLEXION (TIBIALIS ANTICUS)	INVERSION (TIBIALIS ANTICUS)	
L-5	EXTENSION (GLUTEUS MAXIMUS)	FLEXION (MEDIAL HAMSTRINGS)	DORSI-FLEXION (EXT. DIGITORUM COMMUNIS AND EXTENSOR HALLUCIS LONGUS)	EVERSION (PERONEAL MUSCLES)	
S-1	EXTENSION (GLUTEUS MAXIMUS)	FLEXION (LATERAL HAMSTRINGS)	PLANTAR-FLEXION (TRICEPS SURAE)	EVERSION (PERONEAL MUSCLES)	EXTENSION (TOE EXTENSOR MUSCLES)
S-2	EXTENSION (GLUTEUS MAXIMUS)		PLANTAR-FLEXION (TRICEPS SURAE)		FLEXION (LONG, TOE FLEXORS)
S-3					(TOE INTRINSIC MUSCLES)

Fig. 4-12. Diagram of muscles and their action at lower extremity joints affected in various types of myelomeningocele. Neurosegmental level depends on severity of lesion and leads to varying pathologic conditions, depending on how high in spine the nerve roots are involved. (Redrawn from Tzimas.[28])

cord or cauda equina, usually associated with anomalous development of the vertebrae. The two lateral portions of the spinal cord are separated by an osseous or fibrocartilaginous septum, which is attached anteriorly to one or more vertebral bodies, posteriorly to the dura, and occasionally to the deformed vertebral arches as well. Cohen and Sledge pointed out that the term diastematomyelia refers only to the split in the spinal cord and not to the spike or septum frequently found in the cleft.

The persistent neurenteric canal theory of Bremer is the most appealing and seems to make the most sense of the development of this condition. The importance of diastematomyelia is that it is often associated with serious conditions such as congenital scoliosis. If diastematomyelia is unrecognized and the patient has severe scoliosis, any form of traction treatment for the correction of the scoliosis could lead to paraplegia from traction on the tethered spinal cord. The fibrocartilaginous spike or septum can, in effect, act as a thumbtack holding the spinal cord and prevent the cord's normal ascent and migration upward in the spinal canal. Therefore, serious neurological defects such as Arnold-Chiari syndrome can occur. Although most cases of diastematomyelia are diagnosed in childhood, many of them reach adulthood, and the examining physician should be aware of this condition or the opportunity for diagnosis can be missed.

In a series of 20 cases recently described by the author, the oldest patient was 53 years old upon discovery, while the youngest patient was 1 year old. Many cases were diagnosed purely because of a lower-extremity condition, such as cavus of the forefoot, varus of the heel, or calf atrophy. As previously mentioned, all cases of lower-extremity pathology in children should immediately stimulate the examining physician to look upward toward the spine to make the diagnosis. Figure 4-13 shows a child with a typical hairy patch on her back near the lumbar region. Any cutaneous manifestation such as a hair tuft, hemangioma, skin dimple, or other type of external sign should arouse suspicion of an underlying spinal anomaly. In the same illustration, note the patient's right leg, which shows atrophy of the calf and a varus heel. These were the presenting complaints when the patient was first seen.

In 1950 Neuhauser and associates described the roentgenographic findings in diastematomyelia, and in conjunction with Matson and coworkers they gathered a series of patients in whom accurate diagnoses were made preoperatively. Widening of the neural canal in a fusiform fashion is the hallmark of diastematomyelia (Fig. 4-14).

Simril and Thurston published data on the range of normal interpedicular distances. In diastematomyelia, the pedicles adjoining the widened canal are not narrowed or eroded as with an expanding intraspinal tumor. However Cowie pointed out that occasionally the pedicles are flattened next to the widened spinal canal. In addition to the widened spinal canal, almost invariably some degree of spina bifida is found. Other spinal anomalies seen are defects (such as hemivertebra), failures of segmentation (such as congenital bars or block vertebra), or, occasionally, a "butterfly" vertebra in which the posterior spinal elements resemble the wings of a butterfly.

Diastematomyelia can be associated with symptoms ranging from mild backaches to paraplegia. Some patients have no symptoms for years, whereas others have severe lower-extremity deficiency. Normally, during development of the fetus from the 3-month stage to birth, the conus medullaris moves from the tip of the coccyx to the upper border of the third lumbar vertebra. Because the spinal column continues to grow more rapidly than the cord, the level of the cord moves upward to the upper border of the second lumbar vertebra by the age of 5, and it usually remains there or slightly higher thereafter (Fig. 2-4). Any form of traction during active growth or during orthopedic treatment for spinal conditions could cause a traction phenomenon to exert itself on the spine with resulting paraplegia. A complete myelogram is therefore essential in evaluating

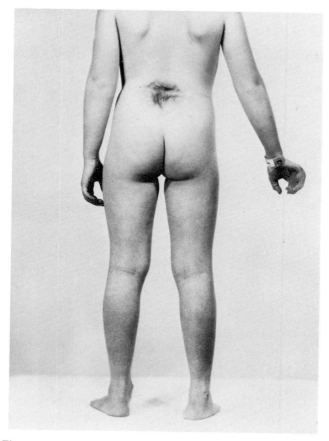

Fig. 4-13. 11-year old girl with congenital hair patch in low
lumbar region. Patient had diastematomyelia and varus deformity
of right foot and ankle, which was the presenting complaint.

the adolescent with lower-extremity problems or spinal evidence of congenital
anomalies (Fig. 4-15).

The treatment of diastematomyelia is neurological excision of the bony or
fibrocartilaginous septum. The mere presence of diastematomyelia in a fully
grown patient is not necessarily a cause for surgical excision. However,
because spinal growth is still remaining in the adolescent, most neurosurgeons
agree that the septum should be removed to prevent future problems (Fig.
4-16). If any type of spinal traction procedure or a spine fusion is necessary, it
should be done at a second stage and not when the diastematomyelia is excised.

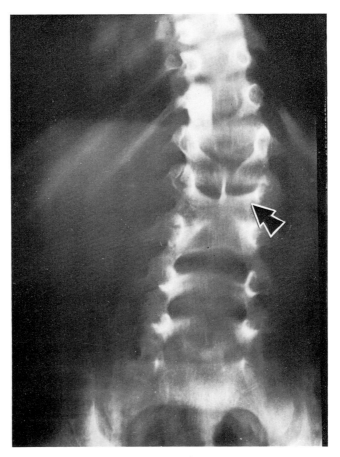

Fig. 4-14. Tomogram of bony spike extending from body of L-2 directly to neural arch of that vertebra. Spike represents diastematomyelia and was tethering patient's spinal cord. Note widened interpedicular distances throughout lumbar region. (From Keim HA: Scoliosis: embryology and anatomy, in The American Academy of Orthopaedic Surgeons: Instructional Course Lectures, vol. XXIV, St. Louis, Mosby, 1975.)

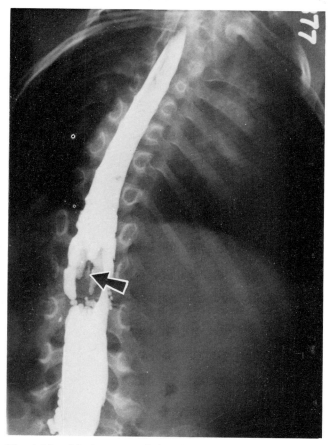

Fig. 4-15. Myelogram outlining diastematomyelia, with a bony
spike at L-2. (From Keim HA: Scoliosis: embryology and
anatomy, in The American Academy of Orthopaedic Surgeons:
Instructional Course Lectures, vol. XXIV, St. Louis, Mosby,
1975.)

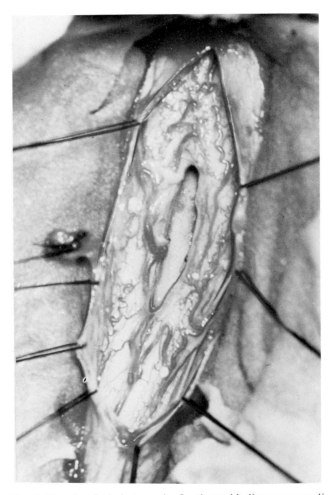

Fig. 4-16. Surgical photograph of patient with diastematomyelia at T-12. Fibrocartilaginous spike splits spinal cord on both sides and exerts a tethering effect. Upon release of this spike, cord ascended almost 2 cm.

REFERENCES

1. Banola A: Surgical treatment of Klippel-Feil syndrome. J Bone Joint Surg 38B:440, 1956
2. Bellamy R, Lieber A, Smith S: Congenital spondylolisthesis of the sixth cervical vertebra. J Bone Joint Surg 56A:405–407, 1974
3. Bentley JFR, Smith JR: Developmental posterior enteric remnants and spinal malformations. The split notochord syndrome. Arch Dis Child 35:76–86, 1960
4. Bertolotti M: Contributo alla conoscenza dei vizii di differenziozione regionale del raclide con speziale della assimilazione della 5ta lumbare. Radiol Med May-June, 1917
5. Bligh AS: Diastematomyelia. Clin Radiol 12:158–163, 1961
6. Bremer JL: Dorsal intestinal fistula; accessory neurenteric canal; diastematomyelia. Arch Pathol 54:132–138, 1952
7. Cameron AH: The Arnold-Chiari and other neuroanatomical malformations associated with spina bifida. J Pathol 73:195, 1957
8. Campbell JB: Congenital anomalies of the neural axis. Surgical management based on embryologic considerations. Am J Surg 75:231–256, 1948
9. Capener CJ: Spondylolisthesis. Br J Surg 19:374, 1931
10. Casolo G: Clinical and roentgenological study of sacralization of the 5th lumbar. Radiol Med Milan 11:357, 1924
11. Chiari H: Ueber veranderungen des kleinbirns infolge von hydrocephalie des grossbirns. Dtsch Med Wochenschr 17:1, 172, 1891
12. Cohen J, Sledge CB: Diastematomyelia . An embryological interpretation with report of a case. Am J Dis Child 100:257–263, 1960
13. Cowie TN: Diastematomyelia with vertebral column defects. Observations on its radiological diagnosis. Br J Radiol 24:156–160, 1951
14. Cowie TN: Diastematomyelia: tomography in diagnosis. Br J Radiol 25:263–266, 1952
15. Hensinger RN, Lang JE, MacEwen GD: Klippel-Feil syndrome. A constellation of associated anomalies. J Bone Joint Surg 56A:1246–1253, 1974
16. James CCM, Lassman LP: Spinal dysraphism. The diagnosis and treatment of progressive lesions in spina bifida occulta. J Bone Joint Surg 44B:828–840, 1962
17. Keim HA, Greene AF: Diastematomyelia and scoliosis. J Bone Joint Surg 55A:1425–1435, 1973
18. Kilian HF: Schilderungen neuer Beckenformen und ihres Verhattens im Leben. Mannheim, Verlag von Bassermann & Mathy, 1834
19. Klippel M, Feil A: Un cas d'absence des vertebres cervicales. Nouvelle Iconographie de la Salpetriere 25:223, 1912
20. Krenz J, Troup JDG: The structure of the pars interarticularis of the lower lumbar vertebrae and its relation to the etiology of spondylolisthesis. J Bone Joint Surg 55B:735–745, 1973
21. Matson DD, Woods RP, Campbell JB, et al: Diastematomyelia (congenital clefts of the spinal cord). Diagnosis and surgical treatment. Pediatrics 6:98–112, 1950
22. Neuhauser EDB, Wittenborg MH, Dehlinger K: Diastematomyelia. Transfixation of the cord or cauda equina with congenital anomalies of the spine. Radiology 54:659–664, 1950

23. Newman PH, Stone KH: The etiology of spondylolisthesis. J Bone Joint Surg 45B:39–59, 1963
24. Patten BM: Embryological stages in the establishing of myeloschisis with spina bifida. Am J Anat 93:365, 1953
25. Sharrard WJW: The mechanism of paralytic deformity in spina bifida. Dev Med Child Neurol 4:310, 1962
26. Shorey WD: Diastematomyelia associated with dorsal kyphosis producing paraplegia. J Neurosurg 12:300–305, 1955
27. Simril WA, Thurston D: The normal interpediculate space in the spines of infants and children. Radiology 64:340–347, 1955
28. Tzimas NA: Orthopaedic care of the child with spina bifida, in Swinyard CA (ed): Comprehensive Care of the Child with Spina Bifida Manifesta. New York, Institute of Rehabilitation Medicine, New York University, 1966, pp 45–65
29. Von Lackum HL: The lumbosacral region: an anatomical study and some clinical observations. J Am Med Assoc 82:1109, 1904
30. Willis TA: The separate neural arch. J Bone Joint Surg 13:709, 1931
31. Wiltse LL: The etiology of spondylolisthesis. J Bone Joint Surg 44A:539, 1962
32. Wiltse LL, Widell EH, Jackson DW: Fatigue fracture: the basic lesion in isthmic spondylolisthesis. J Bone Joint Surg 57A:17–22, 1975
33. Winter RB: Diastematomyelia and spina bifida scoliosis, in Keim HA (ed): First Annual Postgraduate Course on the Management and Care of the Scoliosis Patient. Warsaw, Indiana, Zimmer, 1969, pp 67–69
34. Zachary RB, Sharrard WJW: Spinal dysraphism. Postgrad Med J 43:731, 1967

5
Tumors in the Adolescent Spine

Tumors in the adolescent spine are fortunately almost always benign. Malignant tumors in the adolescent spine are rare, and when they occur, they are usually due to metastatic conditions arising from long bones.

In this chapter the main bony tumors that can involve the adolescent spine are outlined, and some neural tumors—both extradural and intradural—that can also cause severe spinal problems are discussed.

The cells of the muscles and skeleton all share a common "mesodermal" origin but have differentiated to become osteoblasts, osteoclasts, chondroblasts, firbroblasts, and myeloblasts. Although no classification of bone tumors can be totally complete, the most up-to-date classification seems to be that of Aegerter and Kirkpatrick. In their classification, primary lesions are classified as osteogenic, chondrogenic, collagenic, and myelogenic. They describe reactive lesions (which are not true neoplasms), hamartomas (which may be considered benign neoplasms), and true neoplasms (some which are potentially and others which are frankly malignant).

Classification of Bone Tumors (Aegerter and Kirkpatrick, 1968)

I.   Reactive bone lesions
   A.   Osteogenic
      1.   Osteoid osteoma
      2.   Benign osteoblastoma
   B.   Collagenic

     1.   Nonosteogenic fibroma
     2.   Subperiosteal cortical defect
II.   Hamartomas affecting bone
   A.   Osteogenic
     1.   Osteoma
     2.   Osteochondroma
   B.   Chondrogenic
     1.   Enchondroma
   C.   Collagenic
     1.   Angioma (hemangioma)
     2.   Aneurysmal bone cyst
III.   True neoplasms of bone
   A.   Osteogenic
     1.   Osteosarcoma
     2.   Parosteal sarcoma
     3.   Osteoclastoma
   B.   Chondrogenic
     1.   Benign chondroblastoma
     2.   Chondromyxoid fibroma
     3.   Chondrosarcoma
   C.   Collagenic
     1.   Fibrosarcoma
     2.   Angiosarcoma
   D.   Myelogenic
     1.   Plasma cell myeloma
     2.   Ewing's tumor
     3.   Reticulum cell sarcoma
     4.   Hodgkin's disease

The classification listed above is fortunately limited in the adolescent skeleton. A few of the major conditions that can involve the adolescent age group will be described.

OSTEOID OSTEOMA

Osteoid osteoma is a small circumscribed lesion usually no larger than 2 cm in diameter. In the spine, it is generally located in the posterior elements or pedicles of the vertebrae. The osteoid osteoma is characterized (1) clinically, by severe nocturnal pain, out of proportion to its size; (2) radiologically, by a translucent lesion surrounded by a large zone of sclerosis; and (3) pathologically, by a nidus of osteoid surrounded by a network of fine new bone in a vascular fibrous matrix.

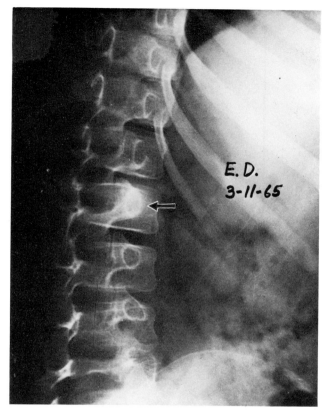

Fig. 5-1.   Osteoid osteoma of the pedicle of 2nd lumbar vertebra,
oblique view. In this "Scottie dog" shadow, cataract can be seen in
dog's eye. Posterior elements of spinal column are most commonly
involved in osteoid osteomas of the spine.

Jaffe was the first to recognize osteoid osteoma as a distinct clinical entity
when he described 5 cases in 1935. At the New York Orthopaedic Hospital
over the last 25 years, 97 cases of osteoid osteoma have been described in the
spine; most of these were found in adolescents (Fig. 5-1). For some unknown
reason, the pain caused by the lesion is classically relieved by aspirin. Osteoid
osteoma is a self-limiting lesion and usually burns itself out after several years;
however, the relief from excisional surgery is so dramatic that surgical excision
is the preferred form of treatment.

Osteoid osteomas can easily masquerade under many types of conditions,
and frequently a patient has scoliosis and gives no history typical of osteoid
osteoma. This makes diagnosis difficult, and the physician must be aware of
these lesions when he examines the adolescent spine. A tipoff is that sometimes

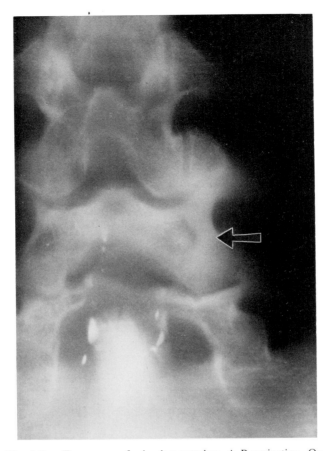

Fig. 5-2.   Tomogram of a lumbar vertebra, A-P projection. Osteoid osteoma, vertebral pedicle has a central opaque nidus surrounded by an area of radiolucency. Tomograms are extremely
helpful in localizing spinal bone tumors.

the patient's supine x-ray shows a greater scoliotic curve than the erect film.
This is due to increasing pain and muscle spasm in the supine position.
Tomograms of the affected area are always helpful in ruling out this diagnosis,
and when the condition is suspected but not proven by x-rays, the patient should
be reexamined at 3-month intervals until the diagnosis is confirmed or totally
ruled out (Fig. 5-2). When the tumor is excised, x-rays in the operating room
are essential. The bony lesion should be removed in toto if possible and an x-ray
taken of the excised specimen to be sure that all of the lesion has been removed.

Osteoid osteomas are twice as common in men than in women, and they
most commonly affect people between ages 10 and 26. In the author's series,
several patients were treated under a misdiagnosis for months and even years

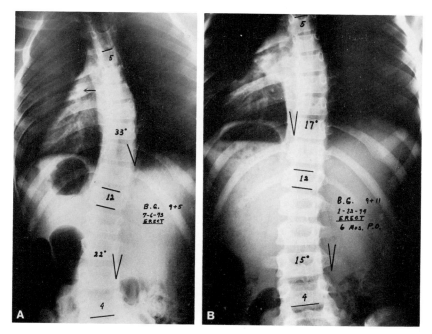

Fig. 5-3*A*. Rare case of osteoid osteoma in the neck of left rib where rib articulates with spine. Tumor produced 33° right thoracic scoliosis because of the severe pain it generated. *B*. Postoperative x-ray 6 months after resection of entire lesion with marked resolution of scoliosis. Pain relief was immediate, and spine straightened completely within 1 year of excisional surgery.

before the correct diagnosis was made. In cases of scoliosis due to osteoid osteoma, most scoliotic curves resolve spontaneously after the tumor has been removed (Fig. 5-3). In some cases it is necessary to apply a Milwaukee brace, since structural curves are relatively permanent due to muscle spasm that persisted for months or years before diagnosis.

The term giant osteoid osteoma has been used to designate an osteoid-forming lesion that is larger than the osteoid osteoma. This lesion is generally considered to be an entirely separate entity from true osteoid osteoma and belongs in a category of benign osteoblastoma. The exact relationship of these two lesions still remains somewhat clouded.

BENIGN OSTEOBLASTOMA

Fortunately, the benign osteoblastoma (giant osteoid osteoma) is relatively uncommon. In the series of Aegerter and Kirkpatrick there were only 18 cases, but the lesions occurred most frequently between the ages of 10 and 25, with the youngest patient being 6, and the oldest 38. The most common site of involvement was in the neural arch of the vertebral column, and 10 of the 18 cases arose in the vertebral axis—8 of them in males and 9 of these between the ages of 8 and 28.

The benign osteoblastoma also causes pain, and in Aegerter's series the type of pain was not much different from that of osteoid osteoma. In fact, in one case, relief with aspirin was dramatic. The benign osteoblastoma is usually not much larger than the osteoid osteoma, but is generally greater than 10 cm in diameter. It is a very destructive lesion and generally replaces an area of bone that has been destroyed. Although there is some sclerosis of surrounding bone, it does not provoke the sclerosis seen in osteoid osteomas. Also, the benign osteoblastoma tends to penetrate bone and sometimes is surrounded by a small soft tissue tumor mass (Fig. 5-4). It has been known to cause severe radiating back pain with paresthesias and paraplegia. The treatment is curettage or local resection in a long bone, but en block excision, if possible, around the spinal canal.

ANGIOMA (HEMANGIOMA)

Hemangiomas are the most common of all benign tumors of the vertebrae. In a study at Schmorl's Institute, Junghanns examined 3829 spinal columns and found 409 hemangiomas—an incidence of 10.7 percent of all spines. Of the 409 cases studied, 579 hemangiomas were counted: 32 of these were in the cervical spine, 350 in the thoracic spine, 107 in the lumbar spine, and 27 in the sacrum. Symptomatic hemangiomas can occur in any bone but are rare outside of the vertebrae and skull. They are almost always found in children and adolescents, and they can have massive involvement of the vertebral body leading to eventual collapse and pressure on the spinal cord and nerve roots. The pattern of bone destruction with characteristic coarse, vertical striations is generally diagnostic in roentgenograms. The vertebral body is usually ballooned in the side-to-side diameter and narrowed in height.

Because of the highly vascular nature of these tumors, surgical excision is extremely dangerous and massive hemorrhage is likely. Hemangiomas are vulnerable to irradiation, which is generally how they are treated.

ANEURYSMAL BONE CYST

Aneurysmal bone cysts have been reported only since 1950 but may have been reported previously under other names. The tumor is a collagenous hamartoma and is benign; because of its balloonlike expansion and multicystic nature, it can be of considerable size and cause displacement symptoms with

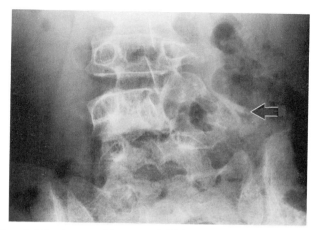

Fig. 5-4.Benign osteoblastoma of 4th lumbar vertebra that caused extreme destruction and erosion of vertebra, with soft tissue displacement and neural involvement. Tumor had to be excised three times before pressure symptoms were completely relieved.

pressure on the spinal cord and nerve roots. An aneurysmal bone cyst generally involves the vertebral bodies and pedicles of the spine. It almost always starts within cancellous or medullary tissue and erodes the cortex from within. The process is a slow, continuous erosion, with bony apposition on the outside causing an expanding lesion to develop.

The main symptom of an aneurysmal bone cyst is pain, most likely due to pressure on surrounding structures and periosteum. The most consistent microscopic finding is a dramatic display of multinucleated giant cells that can

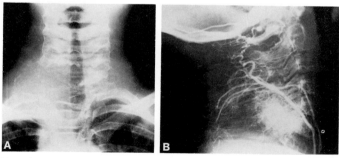

Fig. 5-5A.   Aneurysmal bone cyst in cervical spine showing effects of severe erosion of lower 2 cervical vertebrae. Neurological involvement was severe. B. Angiogram showing blood vessel filling within tumor. Tumor eventually resolved after multiple embolization of all feeder vessels that occluded its blood supply. (Courtesy Sadek Hilal, M.D.)

confuse the pathologist since they resemble "giant cell tumor" or the brown tumor of a parathyroid adenoma.

The treatment for aneurysmal bone cysts is rarely surgical since these lesions are so vascular and cause considerable bleeding. However, cases have been reported of total en block excision of entire vertebral bodies with implantation of large bony struts. X-ray treatment is generally not recommended, although it has been used to thrombose and sclerose the vascular channels supplying the tumor. Figure 5-5 shows an aneurysmal bone cyst that destroyed the cervical spine in a 14-year-old child. The lesion was embolized using small silastic balls injected through the "feeder" vessels. The blood supply to the tumor was halted and the lesion regressed. A surgical approach to this area would have been extremely difficult and dangerous.

HISTIOCYTOSIS "X"

Although histiocytoses are reticuloendothelial disturbances and are not true bone tumors, they are presented here along with true tumors of the spine because of their typical x-ray involvement. The confusion surrounding the histiocytosis X group of conditions has still not been completely delineated, but the condition is definitely one of the reticuloendothelial system and includes Hand-Schüller-Christian disease, eosinophilic granuloma, and Letterer-Siwe disease. All of these conditions are thought to be manifestations of the same process with the eosinophilic granuloma being the mildest form and Letterer-Siwe disease the most malignant and fulminating form of the condition. The main disturbance is in cholesterol metabolism, and the disease is basically metabolic. Only eosinophilic granuloma is described here since this causes such distinct spinal lesions with focal areas of bone destroyed by a granulomatous process of unknown etiology.

Eosinophilic granuloma is almost always seen in childhood and adolescence, and there is a considerable male predominance. In more than half of the cases there are two or more lesions. The most common site is in the frontal bones of the skull, although the lesions have been described in every bone of the skeleton and can involve the vertebrae, where they cause severe flattening of the vertebral bodies.

In the skull and long bones, the radiographic picture of eosinophilic granuloma is usually that of a round or oval radiolucent defect that has no surrounding sclerosis and appears punched out. There is no bony reaction to the destructive process, and flat bones are more frequently involved than cylindrical bones.

When a vertebral body is involved, it collapses dramatically and sometimes gives the appearance of a thin dense plate (Fig. 5-6). The intervertebral

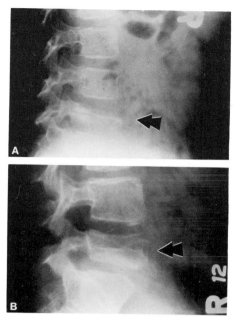

Fig. 5-6*A*. Eosinophilic granuloma of lumbar spine in a 14-year-old child. *B*. Same vertebrae 8 months after original diagnosis. Note restitution of height of 5th lumbar vertebra. However, it will never reach its original height. In eosinophilic granuloma of spine, disc spaces remain normal width, even though vertebral body may collapse to a thin wafer.

discs above and below maintain their normal width, and after normal healing, the vertebral body tends to resume part of its original height. In the vertebral bodies healing usually starts at the periphery and proceeds centrally, and the spine must be protected from further vertebral collapse during remineralization.

MALIGNANT BONE TUMORS

Fortunately, malignant bony tumors in the adolescent are extremely rare. Primary osteosarcomas almost never arise directly in the spine, since they have a predilection for long bones. They are most common in the 10 to 20-year-old age group but rarely arise primarily in vertebrae; they are occasionally found in the flat bones of the pelvis. However, metastatic osteosarcomas are much more common in the adolescent spine and usually are found during the terminal stages of this disease. Junghanns claims that only about 1 percent of all bony sarcomas originate in the spine. Chondrosarcomas, fibrosarcomas, and osteosarcomas are much less common than Ewing tumors and reticulum cell sarcomas. The main malignant tumors in childhood and adolescence are Ewing's tumor, neuroblastoma, and Wilms' tumor.

Ewing's Tumor

Ewing's tumor is a rapidly growing malignant neoplasm that arises from primitive cells of the bone marrow in the young. It is the third most common primary malignant neoplasm of bone, being exceeded only by plasma cell myeloma and osteosarcoma. Like osteosarcoma, Ewing's tumor develops in children, adolescents, and young adults, and most commonly is present in the femur, tibia, and upper extremities. It is rarely found in the spine except after advanced stages of the disease.

Ewing's tumor generally causes severe systemic manifestations, and products of its degeneration enter the bloodstream and produce fever, elevated sedimentation rate, and an increased white blood cell count. The principal presenting complaint is usually pain, and a soft tissue mass is often palpable. By the time a child develops spinal metastases of Ewing's tumor the prognosis is extremely grave, and generally little treatment can be offered. The mortality within the first 4 years of diagnosis is approximately 95 percent regardless of treatment—even radical amputation of an extremity.

Neuroblastoma

Neuroblastoma is a metastasing tumor to the spine that originates in the adrenal medulla or other sympathetic nervous tissue in the child. Multiple lesions are seen, usually in the skull, pelvis, and shafts of long bones. Neuroblastoma may easily simulate Ewing's tumor radiologically and pathologically. When involving the spine, it causes lytic areas and rapidly destroys vertebrae. The tumor is usually fatal.

Neuroblastoma generally spreads through the lymphatic and hematogenous route with severe multiple bony metastases of an osteolytic nature and a small amount of reactive new bone formation. Cranial bones can be severely involved; however, the skeleton is also often the site of metastatic lesions. An aid in diagnosing neuroblastoma is an elevation in catecholamine levels and the metabolic products of catecholamines, such as 3-methoxy4-hydroxymandelic acid (VMA), or homovanillic acid (HVA) in the urine.

Treatment of neuroblastoma almost always consists of surgical excision with postoperative irradiation, combined with chemotherapeutic agents such as vincristine and cyclophosphamide.

Wilms' Tumor

Wilms' tumor is a severe kidney tumor usually seen in infants and children. Treatment consists of total nephrectomy followed by irradiation and actinomycin D therapy. Metastatic involvement of the skeleton is common, and because patients with Wilms' tumor and neuroblastomas receive x-ray treatment, severe spinal deformities due to vertebral growth disturbances many times occur during adolescence. Irradiation therapy for these tumors destroys the vertebral end plates on the side of the tumor. Compensatory unilateral overgrowth on the opposite side leads to severe kyphotic and scoliotic deformities during the adolescent growth years (Fig. 8-19).

NEURAL TUMORS IN THE ADOLESCENT

Most neural tumors involving the adolescent spine are classified as extradural or intradural. The extradural tumors include such benign conditions as hemangioma or fibroblastoma. Intradural tumors are further divided into extramedullary, which involve the meninges (such as meningioma and neurofibroma), and intramedullary tumors (such as ependymoma or astrocytoma).

Extradural Tumors

The extradural hemangioma often is associated with a cutaneous manifestation. A hair tuft can indicate conditions such as diastematomyelia, and cutaneous hemangiomas many times also point to underlying intraspinal pathology. Figure 5-7 illustrates this. The patient had a cutaneous hemangioma that "blushed" when she performed a Valsalva maneuver, so her physician performed a complete neurological investigation and a myelogram. An intraspinal extradural hemangioma was diagnosed, but suspicion had been provoked initially by the cutaneous hemangioma.

Extradural tumors usually are benign and rarely cause serious adolescent difficulty. Intradural lesions, however, can cause severe problems. Meningiomas are intradural extramedullary tumors arising from the meninges. They can enlarge and cause pressure effects on the spinal cord and nerve roots. In these cases local excision usually solves the problem. The most common and serious type of intradural extramedullary tumor is neurofibromatosis.

Neurofibromatosis: Intradural Extramedullary

Neurofibromatosis, or von Recklinghausen's disease, is a hereditary, often congenital, condition involving the supporting tissues of the nervous system both centrally and peripherally. Aegerter classifies this condition as a

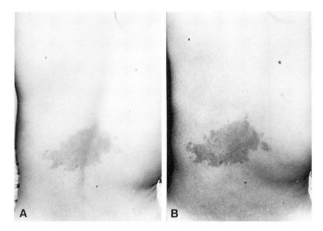

Fig. 5-7. Cutaneous hemangioma in spine of a 13-year-old girl.
A. Resting state with normal color of hemangioma. *B*. After patient
holds her breath and pushes against resistance (Valsalva maneuver), hemangioma blushes. This cutaneous lesion indicated a
more serious problem —intraspinal neoplasm—inside neural canal.

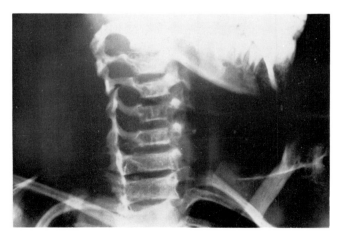

Fig. 5-8. Multiple neurofibromata in cervical spine. Cervical foramina are markedly
enlarged where "dumbbell" lesions caused a pressure effect on bone. (Courtesy Babies
Hospital, Radiology Department, New York City.)

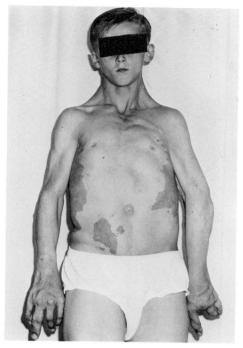

Fig. 5-9.   Neurofibromatosis in a 15-year-old boy. Ring finger of
right hand shows severe hyperthrophy. Middle finger of left hand
has been amputated previously because of marked overgrowth.
Many café-au-lait spots are on chest and abdomen.

skeletal dysplasia, but since it so often causes tumorlike invasion of the spine in
the adolescent, we include it here.

Neurofibromatosis almost always involves the skin but can invade the
skeleton. It can also cause disturbances in other systems such as the endocrine
system and gastrointestinal tract. Kölliker first described neurofibromatosis in
1862, but it was not until 1882 that von Recklinghausen associated the lesions
with the nervous system and the disease took on his name.

Neurofibromatosis involves mainly the nervous system, where groups of
spindle cells arise from either the Schwann or fibrous supportive cells along the
course of peripheral nerves in branches of both the autonomic nervous system
and the meninges. These tumors are pale, moderately firm, and involve
segments and occasionally the entire length of the spinal cord. The diameter of
the nerve trunk is greatly increased and causes pressure on the spinal cord due to
excessive growth in a confined region. Glial tumors within the brain cause
severe cranial damage and can lead to death. The neurofibromas spread along

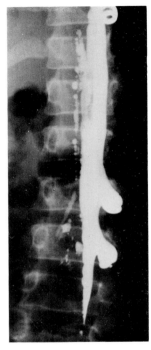

Fig. 5-10. Myelogram of lumbar spine shows a filling defect of dye in pockets produced by neurofibromas. This classical picture is rarely confused with other lesions. (Courtesy Babies Hospital, Radiology Department, New York City.)

the spinal nerve roots and cause bony changes in the vertebrae by direct erosion (Fig. 5-8).

Patients almost always develop café-au-lait spots measuring from several millimeters to many centimeters in diameter. Neurologists claim that any patient having more than five café-au-lait spots over several centimeters in diameter is diagnosed as having neurofibromatosis unless proven otherwise. Since changes in the cranial nerves can occur, the eyes of patients with neurofibromatosis should be examined to rule out optic neuromas. In the skeleton, neurofibromatosis can cause extremely severe forms of scoliosis and is usually associated with a short, sharp, angular curve. (This will be discussed in greater detail in the section on scoliosis.)

Local giantism, or skeletal enlargement, is sometimes most bizarre in neurofibromatosis and can develop in half of the body. The hypertrophy can involve a single bone or an entire extremity, causing marked overgrowth and leg length discrepancy that can also lead to spinal instability due to pelvic obliquity (Fig. 5-9). Some authorities claim that as many as 10 percent of neurofibromas undergo malignant transformation during adult life. Therefore, affected patients must have repeated biopsies throughout their life to detect malignant changes in growing lesions.

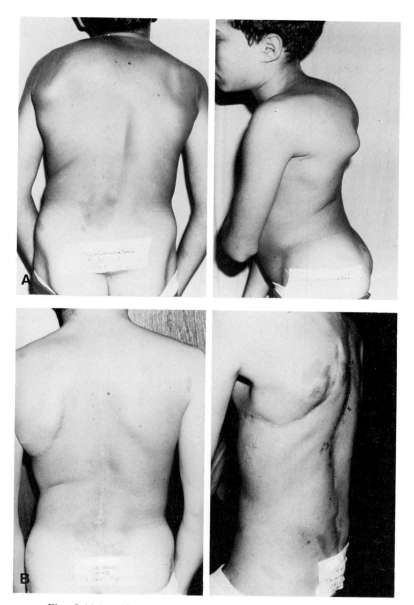

Fig. 5-11*A*.   13-year-old patient with severe kyphoscoliosis of thoracic spine due to neurofibromatosis. *B*. Same patient 2 years after posterior spine fusion and intrathoracic approach through left chest incision to stabilize thoracic spine from in front and help

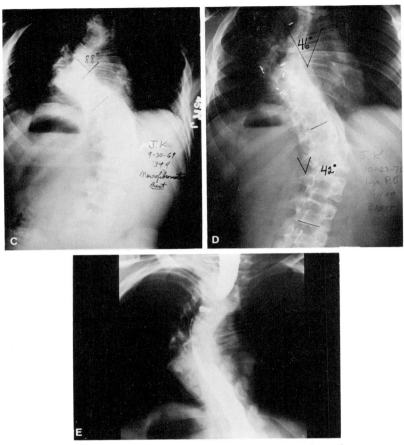

correct kyphosis. *C.* Preoperative x-ray of spine shows short, sharp, angular curve (88°) of neurofibromatosis. *D.* Postoperative x-ray shows thoracic curve reduced to 46°. Neurosurgical clips are result of intraspinal surgery to remove parts of the tumor causing direct spinal cord pressure. *E.* Myelogram shows almost total occlusion of spinal cord due to pressure effects of neurofibromas. Occlusion was relieved neurosurgically.

    Local treatment of neurofibromatosis in the spine consists of correction of any scoliotic or kyphotic deformity and myelographic examination before any treatment (Fig. 5-10) to rule out intraspinal lesions that may become progressive. If intraspinal lesions underlie a spinal fusion, they can cause great difficulties in later life. A patient with symptomatic intraspinal neurofibromas and scoliosis needing surgical correction usually can be treated with a laminec-

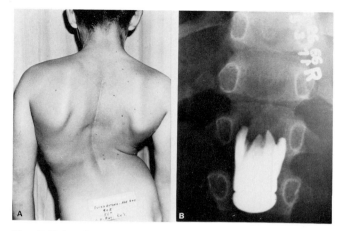

Fig. 5-12A.   9½-year-old boy in whom astrocytoma in middle
thoracic spine was diagnosed at age 2. Excisional surgery and
irradiation treatment had resulted in this structural scoliosis. *B*.
Myelogram of same patient showing intradural intramedullary
tumor with a typical type of "meniscus" effect of myelogram dye.
Widened interpedicular distance in lumbar spine indicates some
type of intraspinal lesion.

tomy and spine fusion at the same stage to remove the tumor and stabilize the
spine (Fig. 5-11).

Intradural Intramedullary Tumors

Intradural intramedullary tumors involve a vast group of benign and
malignant lesions, but most are malignant. These tumors are of interest to the
orthopedic surgeon because they cause severe muscular imbalance around the
spine, leading to scoliosis or kyphosis. If a thorough neurological examination
is not performed at the initial office visit, the tumor can be misdiagnosed and the
patient denied proper treatment. Figure 5-12 shows a patient with an astrocytoma that was present at age 2 but which caused severe deforming changes
in his spine because of cord involvement and scoliotic deformity during
adolescence.

Although most benign neural tumors can be excised locally, malignant
tumors generally lead to progressive changes. Unless they are controlled with
excision or irradiation malignant tumors usually are fatal. Patients with malignant tumors should not be neglected, however, if spinal deformity occurs
because some of them live for many years, and judicious bracing or the use of
plastic corsets can often give them a functional and comfortable life.

REFERENCES

1. Aegerter E, Kirkpatrick J: Orthopaedic Diseases, ed 3. Philadelphia, Saunders, 1968, pp 546–585
2. Cohen J: Simple bone cysts. J Bone Joint Surg 42A:609, 1960
3. Coley B, Lenson N: Osteoid osteoma. Am J Surg 77:3, 1949
4. Compere E, Johnson E, Coventry M: Vertebra plana (Calve's disease) due to eosinophilic granuloma. J Bone Joint Surg 36A:969, 1954
5. Dahlin D, Johnson E: Giant osteoid osteoma. J Bone Joint Surg 36A:559, 1954
6. Golding J: The natural history of osteoid osteoma; with a report of twenty cases. J Bone Joint Surg 36B:218, 1954
7. Jaffe H: Osteoid osteoma. Arch Surg 31:709, 1935
8. Jaffe H, Lichtenstein L: Solitary unicameral bone cyst with emphasis on the roentgen picture, the pathologic appearance and the pathogenesis. Arch Surg 44:1004, 1942
9. Jaffe H: Aneurysmal bone cyst. Bull Hosp Joint Dis 11:3, 1950
10. Jaffe H: Benign osteoblastoma. Bull Hosp Joint Dis 17:141, 1956
11. Keim HA, Reina E: Osteoid osteoma as a cause of scoliosis. J Bone Joint Surg 57A: 159, 1975
12. Lichtenstein L: Aneurysmal bone cyst. Cancer 3:279, 1950
13. MacClellan D, Wilson F: Osteoid osteoma of the spine. J Bone Joint Surg 49A:111, 1967
14. Marsh BW, Bonfiglio M, Brady LP, et al: Benign osteoblastoma: range of manifestations. J Bone Joint Surg 57A:1–9, 1975
15. McCarroll H: Clinical manifestations of congenital neurofibromatosis. J Bone Joint Surg 32A:601, 1950
16. Schmorl G, Junghanns H: The Human Spine in Health and Disease, ed 2. New York, Grune & Stratton, 1971, pp 326–343
17. Scott J: Scoliosis and neurofibromatosis. J Bone Joint Surg 47B:240, 1965
18. Swenson O: Wilms' tumor and neuroblastoma, in Pediatric Surgery. New York, Appleton-Century-Crofts, 1969, p 874
19. von Recklinghausen F: Ueber die multiplen fibrome der haut und ihre beziehung zu den multiplen neuromen. Berlin, August Hirschwald, 1882

6
Trauma and the Adolescent Spine

Because of the adolescent patient's youth, most minor traumatic episodes resolve quickly. Sprains, which are ligamentous injuries, usually heal rapidly, and most adolescents are bothered only by mild aches lasting for a few days. Acute and chronic muscular strains seldom require more than cursory treatment and rarely plague this age group.

The facet syndrome, which commonly affects adults, is actually a subluxation of one facet over another and occurs with improper lifting or twisting maneuvers usually associated with some form of sport or occupation. These, too, rarely cause much trouble in the adolescent.

Fractures in the adolescent are fairly rare, except in cases of extreme violence. When fractures are associated with cervical spine injury and dislocation, consequences can be extremely serious. Since cervical spine fractures will be covered in a separate monograph in this series, they will only be given cursory treatment here. Most cervical spine injuries occur in children because of falls or diving accidents. They rarely result from automobile accident whiplash injuries so common in the adult. Because of the ligamentous laxity in the adolescent, fractures are much less likely to cause transection of the spinal cord in adolescents than in adults. However, treatment is essentially the same in each case—immobilization and reduction of the fracture fragments as promptly as possible with cervical traction and open reduction when indicated.

In the younger adolescent, cervical spine facets occasionally sublux; unilateral dislocation of the cervical facets can be complete, and this usually happens during some form of contact sport when a child's head is twisted to one side and severely rotated. The head usually remains in that position because the

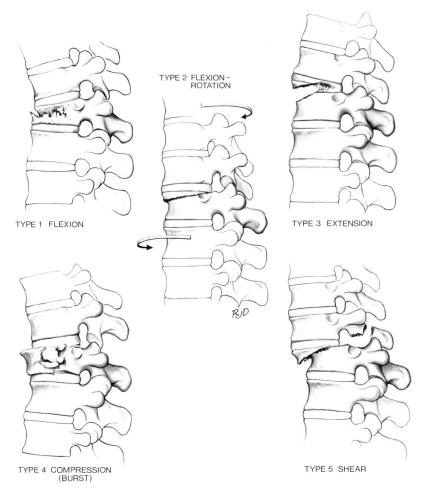

TYPE 1 FLEXION

TYPE 2 FLEXION –
ROTATION

TYPE 3 EXTENSION

TYPE 4 COMPRESSION
(BURST)

TYPE 5 SHEAR

Fig. 6-1.   Holdsworth's classification of spinal trauma (see text).

facets are locked and cannot return to their normal anatomical relationship. Such facet subluxations often are almost impossible to demonstrate on roentgenograms. But if they are suspected, traction usually helps reduce the muscle spasm, and sometimes the facets can be released with gentle manipulation.

An excellent classification of spinal injuries has been formulated by Holdsworth (Fig. 6-1). In his experience with over 1000 patients in all age groups with spinal fractures and neural injuries he postulated that most bony lesions fall into one of five categories, each caused by a specific mechanism.

1. Pure flexion injuries cause a wedge fracture that is almost always stable.

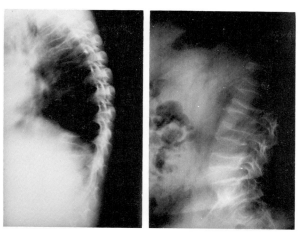

Fig. 6-2. Multiple compression fractures with severe osteoporosis in an 11-year-old boy with advanced asthma. Patient had
received steroid therapy for approximately 2 years and died during
an acute asthmatic crisis 2 weeks after films were taken.

X-rays show compression of the anterior part of the vertebral body usually
wih intact end plates and no significant separation of the spinous processes
(Fig. 6-2).

2. Flexion-rotation injuries produce an unstable fracture dislocation with rupture of the posterior ligament complex, separation of the spinous processes,
   a slice fracture of the upper border of the lower vertebra, and dislocation of
   the lower articular facets of the upper vertebra (Fig. 6-3 A, B).
3. Extension lesions rupture the intervertbral disc and the anterior longitudinal
   ligament and avulse a small bone fragment from the anterior border of the
   dislocated vertebra (teardrop). The dislocation almost always reduces spontaneously and is stable in flexion.
4. Compression injuries ("burst" fractures) result in a fracture of the end plate
   as the nucleus pulposus of the intervertebral disc is forced into the vertebral
   body and causes it to burst with outward displacement of fragments of the
   body. Since the ligaments remain intact, these comminuted fractures are
   stable (Fig. 6-4).
5. Shearing lesions cause forward displacement of the whole vertebra and an
   unstable fracture of the articular processes or pedicles (Fig. 6-5).

Most spinal injuries in the adolescent occur in the thoracolumbar area.
They differ mainly from comparable lesions in the adult because their course is
usually relatively benign and vertebral body height is usually restored during
healing. However, because of growth potential, spinal vertebral deformities

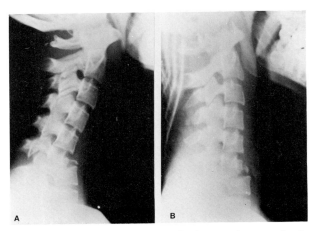

Fig. 6-3A.   Lateral x-ray of severe flexion-rotation-type fracture
dislocation of cervical 6 and 7 in a 13-year-girl. She had immediate
total neurological deficit consisting of almost complete quadriplegia. B. Lateral view showing reduction of fracture after application of skull tongs. Anterior cervical spine fusion was performed to
stabilize cervical spine, and over the next 18 months 80 percent
of all neurological functions returned.

accompany certain types of epiphyseal injuries, especially those in the thoracic
and lumbar region.

In most instances of trauma to the adolescent spine, vehicular accidents,
falls or jumps from heights, and sporting mishaps account for approximately
one-third of all injuries. Hubbard studied 42 consecutive spinal cord injuries in
adolescents and divided them into five different areas on an anatomical basis.
The distribution of the injuries at the different levels showed that two or more
vertebrae were injured in 21 patients, or 50 percent of the series, and 11 cases
(26 percent) had lesions in two or more regions. This illustrates the degree of
trauma that is generally necessary to injure the adolescent spine.

Of the 42 patients, 28 sustained stable fractures of the spinal column,
which in most cases involved the vertebral body. Fractures of the neural arch,
facet, or transverse process accounted for the rest of the stable injuries.
One-third of the patients (14) suffered fracture dislocations, but there were no
joint dislocations or spinal cord injuries without evidence of bony trauma. The
most common mechanism of injury was hyperflexion, which occurred in 23 of
the 42 patients. Of these, 21 had stable, and 2 unstable, spinal injuries. Stable
injuries were seen most frequently in the thoracic region, and unstable lesions
caused by hyperflexion were noted only in the cervical spine.

All the hyperextension injuries were confined to the cervical spine, with 5
of the 6 being unstable. The cervical spine was also most susceptible to vertical

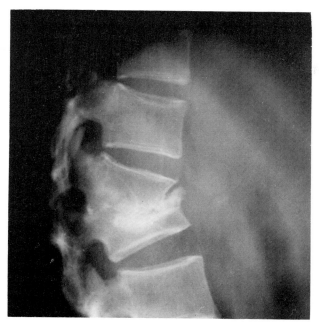

Fig. 6-4.   Severe compression fracture after a fall from a horse. Injury was state and only bedrest and plaster jacket immobilization were required. Vertebral bodies fused spontaneously and little cosmetic deformity remained. There was no neurologic damage at time of injury.

compression, with 3 of the 4 lesions, including the only unstable injury, occurring in this area. Flexion-rotation injuries clustered at the thoracolumbar and upper lumbar levels.

None of the 28 patients with stable spinal injuries had any evidence of neural trauma. Of the 14 patients with unstable lesions, 8 suffered neurological damage, 6 spinal cord damage, and 2 nerve root damage. Neural injury occurred in 4 cases with injuries to the cervical spine; 2 each from forced hyperflexion and hyperextension. There were 4 patients with complete quadriplegia or paraplegia; 2 recovered, 1 improved slightly, and 1 remained completely quadriplegic.

The treatment of these patients involved conservative therapy in all 22 stable spinal injuries with 5 receiving no care at all because the fracture was not recognized. Five of the patients with unstable lesions, all in the cervical spine, were treated nonoperatively. Spinal fusions were performed in 9 patients, combined with laminectomy in 2 cases with neural involvement. The remaining 7 patients received fusions for gross spinal instability. An interesting

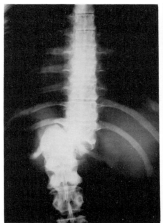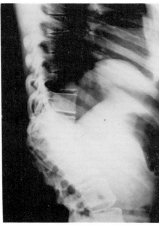

Fig. 6-5.   Severe shearing deformity due to auto accident in which
car hit tree at high speed and patient was thrown from car. She was
not wearing a seatbelt and sustained this severe fracture-dislocation
at junction of thoracic and lumbar spine. She has been totally
paraplegic since injury.

roentgenographic finding was that the height of involved vertebral bodies was
restored in all fractures with follow-up of 6 months or longer. Varying degrees
of repair from partial restitution to bony overgrowth were also observed. The
extent of remodeling in the spine seemed to be directly related to the severity of
the initial injury and the patient's age, with younger individuals showing a
greater ability to restore normal vertebral shape.

Rotary dislocations in the atlantoaxial joint seem to be the most common
lesion in children with injuries to the atlas and axis. Fractures of the odontoid
process are much more frequent in the adult. Injuries in the immature adolescent spine also show a much higher incidence of trauma involving females than
in the adult group, with a greater susceptibility of the thoracic, thoracolumbar,
and lumbar areas. Interestingly, degenerative changes rarely follow adolescent
spinal injuries; however, these may occur much later in life. One finding that is
unique in the adolescent spine after severe spinal trauma is that mild scoliosis
sometimes develops in cases of stable thoracic, thoracolumbar, or lumbar
injury associated with hyperflexion forces.

A kyphotic deformity is usually found in cases of severe vertebral body
collapse and fracture dislocation. Laminectomy without spinal fusion is always
contraindicated in these patients because it leads to gross instability of the
thoracic and lumbar spine, since soft tissues have already been interrupted by
the traumatic force and laminectomy further divides the only stabilizing elements holding the patient's spine together.

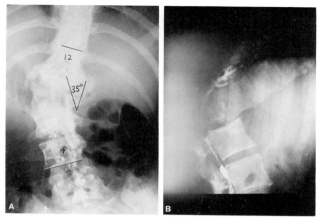

Fig. 6-6. After falling from a 30-foot height, this 15-year-old girl sustained an unstable fracture dislocation at junction of lumbar 1 and 2. A posterior decompressive laminectomy was performed, but no bony fusion was done. Patient obtained no relief from total paraplegia but developed a severe kyphotic deformity because of instability of spine in lumbar region. *B*. 90° angle in lateral plane resulted from lack of bony fusion. Patient developed large skin sores and eventually required anterior and posterior spine fusion for stabilization.

The author has seen many patients with severe kyphotic compression fractures of the vertebral bodies in the thoracolumbar junction. These patients had prompt spinal decompression with a wide laminectomy and no spinal fusion. In all instances the patients' spines gradually "jack-knifed" and caused severe hyperflexion deformities later necessitating major reconstructive procedures. All of these patients required an anterior approach through the chest to prop up the vertebral bodies from in front using a rib-strut graft, followed by a posterior spinal fusion to ensure spinal stability anteriorly and posteriorly.

The only clinical indication for laminectomy in an acute spinal injury is one in which neurological symptoms are progressing while the patient is under observation. Also, in rare instances laminograms reveal a bony spike pressing directly on the spinal cord or nerve roots. In almost all cases of severe spinal trauma causing neurological complications, early operative reduction and stabilization are indicated to prevent further spinal cord damage and kyphotic deformity (Fig. 6-6).

Because of the rapid healing processes in the adolescent, treatment of the milder forms of fractures and dislocations is usually not necessary for more than 2 or 3 months.

Adolescents rarely have spontaneous interbody fusion after severe spinal trauma. This happens quite frequently in adults, but in the adolescent there is so much soft tissue and cartilaginous material at the end plates of the vertebral bodies that growth occurs and bony fusion is rare.

In general, we speak of spinal fractures as being related to compression fractures of the vertebral body, fractures that involve the facet joints, and fractures of the transverse processes. In the thoracic and thoracolumbar regions, compression fractures to the vertebral bodies are extremely common and in most adolescents they are seldom recognized. Compression fractures result from a fall from a tree or some type of minor sport accident to which the adolescent pays little mind, and they heal quickly. Fractures of the transverse processes, uncommon in the adolescent spine, almost always are found in the lumbar region. More commonly, the apophyses of the transverse processes tend to be avulsed because the junction of these apophyses is much weaker than the bony structure of the transverse processes.

As mentioned before, fracture dislocations are generally classified as stable and unstable. The stable types tend to cause mild spinal deformity in later life, but if a great deal of spinal growth remains, they often correct themselves by remodeling. The unstable type of fracture dislocation should always be stabilized since the adolescent is constantly exposed to additional traumatic situations, and leaving a spinal segment unstable only predisposes it to more trouble in the future.

Recently, instrumentation—especially the Harrington type—has been found most useful in stabilizing fracture dislocations around the thoracic and lumbar spine (Fig. 6-7 A-D). The Harrington compression or distraction system can be used; however, the distraction device used on both sides of the spinous processes tends to be the most effective in reducing and stabilizing dislocated vertebrae.

At the time of instrumentation, a wide bilateral-lateral fusion should be performed using autogenous bone, and the patient's spine must be protected with plaster immobilization for at least 6 months after surgery to ensure solid bony union. Many patients treated with this technique are ambulatory much earlier, and neurological return is helped by ensuring a stable and anatomically reduced spine. Whether prompt stabilization actually ensures neurological improvement remains controversial. Nevertheless, almost all authors agree that nursing care and patient management are greatly enhanced with surgical stabilization and early mobilization.

DISC INJURIES IN ADOLESCENCE

Although herniations of the intervertebral disc are really degenerative, they are often associated with trauma in the adolescent. For this reason they are included in this chapter.

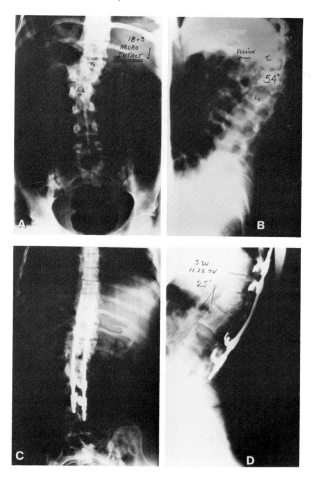

Fig. 6-7 *A,B*.   18-year old girl injured in an auto accident. She had a severe shearing fracture dislocation of T-11, 12, and L-1 (Holdsworth type 5). This unstable fracture was treated by surgical instrumentation and fusion. *C,D*. Compression-type Harrington instrumentation used on both sides of spinous processes. Reduction and stabilization of all fracture fragments have been combined with bilateral-lateral spine fusion using autogenous bone. Note reduction of previous kyphotic deformity. (Courtesy David Bradford, M.D.)

Lumbar intervertebral disc herniations in the adult are extremely common and usually have characteristic clinical findings. However, disc protrusions in adolescents are rare but are common enough to merit special consideration because they are frequently misdiagnosed and improperly treated. In 1969 Bradford and Garcia reviewed 30 patients, 19 men and 11 women, all with surgical treatment for herniations in the lumbar intervertebral disc. Diagnosis was extremely difficult in 14 patients, and 16 patients underwent laminectomy with spinal fusion. The major problem in diagnosing a disc herniation was the examining physician's failure to appreciate the possibility of a herniated disc. The most common misdiagnosis was disc space infection, and some cases were even diagnosed as severe psychiatric conditions. There was a traumatic history of between 30 percent and 60 percent in all cases, and this seems to be generally true in the adult spine as well.

Degenerative ulceration in the intervertebral discs begins early in life. A drop in the water content of the discs from a high of 88 percent in the fetus to 80 percent in a 12-year old and 70 percent in a 70-year old seems to lead to disc degeneration. The protein-polysaccharide fraction of the nucleus pulposus decreases with advancing age, and this decrease seems to lower the water-binding capacity and elasticity of the disc material. Adolescent patients generally complain of pain as their chief symptom when they have a herniated disc. Abnormal neurologic findings are generally rare, and muscle spasm, abnormal straight leg raising, and sciatic-type scoliosis are most common.

In the lumbar region, the fourth and fifth discs are most frequently affected. Traumatic and degenerative changes cause a small tear in the posterior rim of the annulus fibrosus, permitting the softer nucleus pulposus to herniate into the neural canal. Because of direct pressure on and compression of the nerve root, mechanical irritation develops with pain along the dermatome of that root (Fig. 6-8). Additionally, the motor fibers of the affected root are compressed, and this leads to atrophy and weakness in appropriate muscles. Most adolescents complain of severe pain with sciatica developing along the sciatic nerve in the posterolateral thigh and calf. (The sciatic nerve arises from the fourth and fifth lumbar and the first, second, and third sacral nerve roots.)

Pain from a herniated disc is usually centered in the lumbar region with radiation to the buttocks, posterior thigh, calf, and occasionally the foot. The pain often is associated with numbness and paresthesias. In most adolescents, pain is relieved with recumbency and aggravated on assuming routine activities, such as sports. Many times this leads to the diagnosis of malingering by unsympathetic parents and physical education instructors.

Because a disc herniation at each spinal cord level can cause a distinctive picture depending on which nerve root is compressed, one can determine after careful physical examination exactly which disc is involved and which nerve root is being compromised. A clever physician can usually diagnose a disc herniation on the basis of a clinical history and a thorough physical examination. However, when surgery is contemplated, a myelogram is almost always indicated to facilitate diagnosis and localize the level of the herniation. Electrodiagnostic tests, such as nerve conduction studies and electromyography, are also helpful.

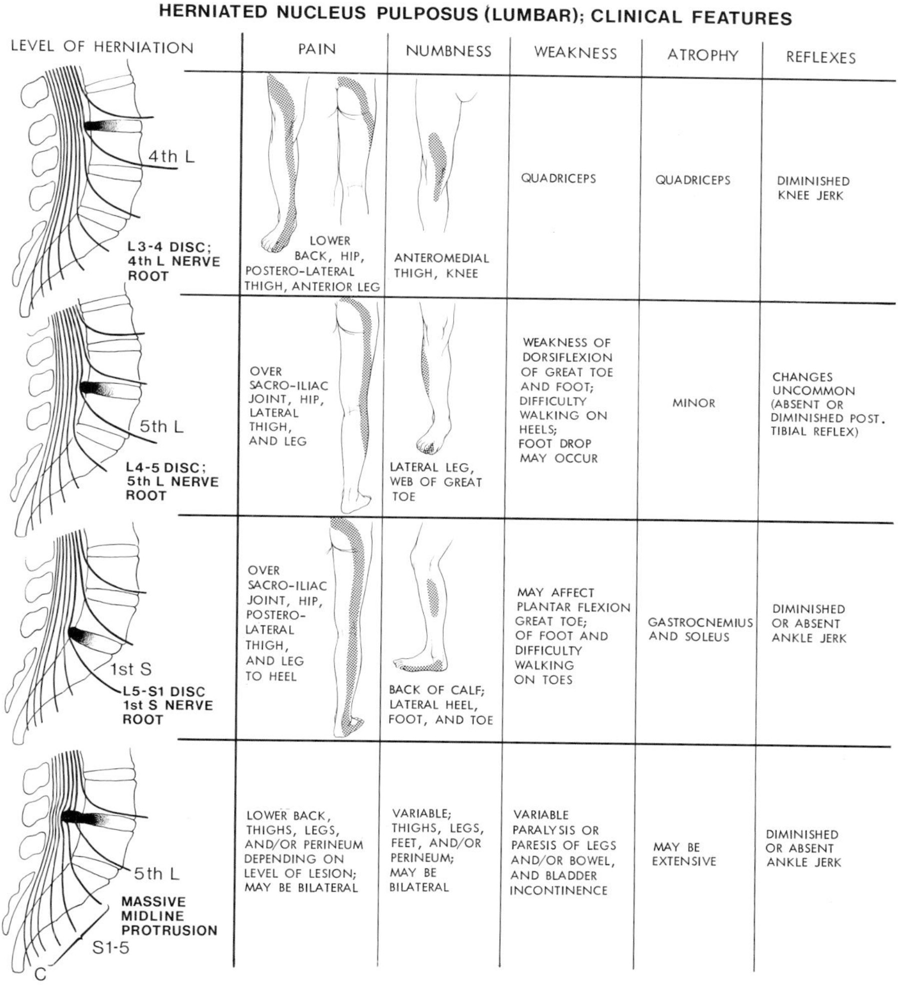

HERNIATED NUCLEUS PULPOSUS (LUMBAR); CLINICAL FEATURES

LEVEL OF HERNIATION	PAIN	NUMBNESS	WEAKNESS	ATROPHY	REFLEXES
4th L — L3-4 DISC; 4th L NERVE ROOT	LOWER BACK, HIP, POSTERO-LATERAL THIGH, ANTERIOR LEG	ANTEROMEDIAL THIGH, KNEE	QUADRICEPS	QUADRICEPS	DIMINISHED KNEE JERK
5th L — L4-5 DISC; 5th L NERVE ROOT	OVER SACRO-ILIAC JOINT, HIP, LATERAL THIGH, AND LEG	LATERAL LEG, WEB OF GREAT TOE	WEAKNESS OF DORSIFLEXION OF GREAT TOE AND FOOT; DIFFICULTY WALKING ON HEELS; FOOT DROP MAY OCCUR	MINOR	CHANGES UNCOMMON (ABSENT OR DIMINISHED POST. TIBIAL REFLEX)
1st S — L5-S1 DISC; 1st S NERVE ROOT	OVER SACRO-ILIAC JOINT, HIP, POSTERO-LATERAL THIGH, AND LEG TO HEEL	BACK OF CALF; LATERAL HEEL, FOOT, AND TOE	MAY AFFECT PLANTAR FLEXION GREAT TOE; OF FOOT AND DIFFICULTY WALKING ON TOES	GASTROCNEMIUS AND SOLEUS	DIMINISHED OR ABSENT ANKLE JERK
5th L — MASSIVE MIDLINE PROTRUSION S1-5	LOWER BACK, THIGHS, LEGS, AND/OR PERINEUM DEPENDING ON LEVEL OF LESION; MAY BE BILATERAL	VARIABLE; THIGHS, LEGS, FEET, AND/OR PERINEUM; MAY BE BILATERAL	VARIABLE PARALYSIS OR PARESIS OF LEGS AND/OR BOWEL, AND BLADDER INCONTINENCE	MAY BE EXTENSIVE	DIMINISHED OR ABSENT ANKLE JERK

Fig. 6-8. Diagram of disc herniations at various levels. (Adapted from original painting by Frank H. Netter, M.D., from Clinical Symposia, copyright Ciba Pharmaceutical Company, Division of Ciba-Geigy Corp. All rights reserved.)

A disc herniation at the third and fourth intervertebral discs characteristically involves the fourth lumbar nerve root. This leads to low back pain with radiation down the posterolateral thigh and anterior leg. There is numbness in the anteromedial thigh and knee with quadriceps muscle weakness and atrophy. The knee reflex is almost always diminished or absent.

A disc herniation at the lumbar four and five levels involves the fifth lumbar nerve root and causes pain over the sacroiliac joint, hip, and lateral thigh and leg. There is loss of sensation over the lateral aspect of the calf and in the great toe web space. Muscle weakness involves the anterior muscles of the lower leg, with weakness in dorsiflexion of the great toe and foot and difficulty in walking on the heels. Atrophy and reflex changes are uncommon. The posterior tibial reflex occasionally is absent.

Herniations of the lumbar disc at the fifth lumbar interspace between lumbar five and the sacrum involve the first sacral nerve root. Herniations cause pain in the sacroiliac joint and down the posterolateral thigh, leg, and heel. Numbness is common in the back of the calf and the lateral side of the foot. Weakness is noted on plantar flexion of the foot and great toe, and the patient has difficulty walking on his toes. The gastrocnemius and soleus muscles are atrophied around the calf, and the ankle jerk reflex is usually absent or diminished.

In the adolescent a massive midline disc protrusion is rare. The protrusion is usually associated with major trauma and can cause the exact symptoms of an intraspinal neoplasm—pain down the entire back of the legs, perineum, and thighs, depending on the location of the midline protrusion. Numbness and weakness are variable, and atrophy is extensive in neglected cases. The ankle jerk is almost always diminished or absent.

Herniated discs are treated best in the adolescent by conservative care, since they occasinally resolve on bedrest and approprate medications. However, in resistant cases laminectomy and excision of the herniated disc are required. Occasionally, chemonucleolysis with chymopapain dissolves the offending disc material. Spinal fusions as a combined procedure do not seem as important in the adolescent as they are in the adult since adolescents rarely have arthritic conditions, and also because laminectomy alone is often successful in adolescents. Fusion is routinely combined with laminectomy in the adolescent only in cases of congenital anomalies involving the same vertebral area, such as sacralization of the transverse process of lumbar five on one side. In this case, a spinal fusion from lumbar four to the sacrum is indicated, along with the removal of a herniated disc at lumbar five and exploration at lumbar four.

Fortunately, traumatic disc herniations in the adolescent are rare. However, when they do occur, prompt recognition and treatment are mandatory to obtain beneficial results.

REFERENCES

1. Blount W: Fractures in Children. Baltimore, Williams & Wilkins, 1955, p 207
2. Bradford D, Garcia A: Herniations of the lumbar intervertebral disc in children and adolescents. A review of thirty surgically treated cases. JAMA 210:2045, 1969

3. Davis A: Injuries of the spinal column, in Instructional Course Lectures. The American Academy of Orthopaedic Surgeons 6. Ann Arbor, Edwards, 1949, p 73

4. Davis L: Treatment of spinal cord injuries. Arch Surg 69:88, 1954

5. Epstein J, Lavine L: Herniated lumbar intervertebral discs in teen-age children. J Neurosurg 21:1070, 1964

6. Holdsworth F: Fractures, dislocations, and fracture dislocations of the spine. J Bone Joint Surg 45B:6, 1953

7. Holdsworth F: Fractures, dislocations, and fracture-dislocations of the spine. J.Bone Joint Surg 52A:1534–1551, 1970

8. Hubbard D: Injuries of the spine in children and adolescents. Clin Orthop 100:56, 1974

9. Key J: Intervertebral-disc lesions in children and adolescents. J Bone Joint Surg 32A:97, 1950

10. Nicoll E: Fractures of the dorsolumbar spine. J Bone Joint Surg 31B:376, 1949

11. Roaf R: A study of the mechanics of spinal injuries. J Bone Joint Surg 42B:810, 1960

12. Webb J, Svien H, Kennedy R: Protruded lumbar intervertebral discs in children. JAMA 154:1153, 1954

7

Infections and Inflammatory Lesions of the Adolescent Spine

Infectious diseases in the adolescent are most often localized in major joints of the extremities. However, the spine occasionally is involved in suppurative osteomyelitis, which can be acute, chronic, or focal (Brodie's abscess). The spine can also be the site of nonsuppurative osteomyelitis in the form of tuberculosis, brucellosis, and different types of fungal infections of bone.

Perhaps the most disturbing form of vertebral inflammation is that involving the disc space in the adolescent. Disc space infections are relatively uncommon in children but always present a diagnostic challenge. Many reports of intervertebral disc infection in children emphasize the relatively benign nature of the conditions, and the problem usually resolves spontaneously but involves difficult diagnostic procedures and major decisions regarding treatment. Disc space infections are generally thought to be caused by an infectious agent, most frequently hemolytic *(Staphylococcus aureus)*. In adults, S. aureus is present in approximately 70 percent of patients. However, in children the organism is difficult to demonstrate, and a specific bacterium is cultured in only a few disc space infections, even after needle and open biopsy of the involved intervertebral disc.

The mode of infection of the intervertebral disc in the adolescent is not quite clear, but it is probably best explained because of anatomical characteristics in this age group. The intervertebral discs of the embryo and child receive nutrition by blood vessels from the surfaces of adjacent vertebral bodies. This allows bacteria to enter the disc tissue hematogenously, which is not possible in the adult. The vascular supply to the intervertebral disc is greater in early life and gradually decreases with advancing age. Another source of intervertebral disc infection is direct innoculation of the bacteria, such as in lumbar puncture or previous surgery.

A child with "discitis," or disc space infection, usually experiences an abrupt onset of malaise, fever, and increasing back pain. The adolescent usually refuses to walk and carries his back in a stiff manner, usually squatting at the knees and hips in order to pick up something. The patient exhibits marked irritability, decreased appetite, and weight loss. When the lumbar spine is involved, the hamstrings are tight and the patient has a positive iliopsoas sign; possible hip joint involvement must then be considered.

Laboratory studies often show an elevated white blood cell count and usually an elevated sedimentation rate. Roentgenographic findings are meager, especially during the first 3 or 4 weeks. Tomograms have sometimes been helpful, especially in establishing a baseline during the early stages of the condition and in providing comparison views 3 to 4 weeks after onset (Fig. 7-1 A-D). Occasionally, the paravertebral shadow widens at the site of involvement, and areas of marginal bone destruction are seen in the vertebrae. Patients are treated empirically and x-rays are repeated at 1- to 2-week intervals until intervertebral disc narrowing at the site of maximum tenderness confirms the diagnosis.

In the differential diagnosis, such conditions as spinal cord tumors, tuberculosis, brucellosis, and salmonellosis must be considered. In the younger adolescent, the initial reduction in disc space height is usually followed in about 3 months by restoration to the normal preinfectious height. In older patients, the disc space may remain narrowed into and throughout adult life.Many times this narrowing culminates in spontaneous fusion between the vertebral bodies.

The treatment for acute disc space infections usually is to rest the spine in recumbency either on a firm bed or in a plaster of paris jacket. This inludes the hips and thighs when the lumbar spine is affected, or the head and neck when the thoracic or cervical spine is involved. Treatment in recumbency is continued until all back pain, muscle spasm, and local tenderness have subsided, and until the patient's temperature, sedimentation rate, and white blood cell count are within normal limits.

An attempt at identifying the causative organism is sometimes justified, especially when the patient is not improving clinically. A closed biopsy using the Craig technique can be done under an image intensifier with relative safety using general anesthesia (Fig. 7-2). Occasionally, the tissue obtained will grow the infecting organism, and proper antibiotic treatment can be started. If the organism cannot be identified, physicians often prefer to treat the patient empirically for an S. aureus infection with appropriate antibiotics. Antibiotics are usually administered for 6 to 8 weeks, and the patient is allowed to assume the erect posture in a plaster body jacket or a spinal brace after all symptoms have resolved. The patient should use this form of back support for 4 to 6

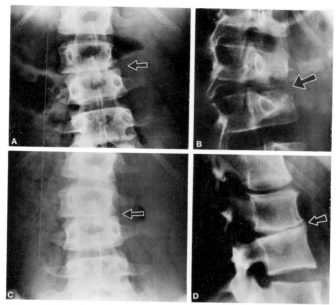

Fig. 7-1   X-rays (taken 3 weeks after onset of symptoms) of a 13-year-old girl with acute onset of low back pain diagnosed as disc space infection. Note irregularity of vertebral bodies between lumbar 2 and 3, with slight subluxation to left between these vertebrae. Oblique view *(B)* shows erosion of inferior body of lumbar 2 and superior body of lumbar 3. *C,D*. X-rays made 6 months after bedrest, antibiotic therapy, and immobilization by body cast. Craig needle biopsy was performed, but no bacteria were isolated. Patient was treated empirically with complete resolution of all symptoms, but permanent disc space narrowing remains.

months until bony healing takes place. If a paravertebral abscess forms and the organism localizes in suppurative areas, it is sometimes appropriate to open and drain the wound and use closed suction-irrigation technique.

Adult pyogenic disc infections differ from those of children in that in the adult the onset is usually more gradual, the course of the disease is slower, and the clinical pattern is more confusing. Because most children are healthy, disc infections are easier to diagnose and treat.

Rocco and Eyring reviewed 155 cases of disc space infection in adolescents and children; 54 percent were girls and 40 percent were adolescents. The most frequently involved levels were lumbar four and five, and the next most frequently involved areas were lumbar three and four. These investigators classified the clinical symptom complexes of these children into five major groups: back symptoms, hip-leg symptoms, meningeal symptoms, abdominal symptoms, and the ''irritable'' child complex. Many cases were initially

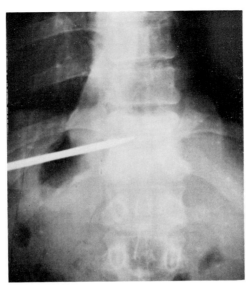

Fig. 7-2   Craig needle biopsy between vertebral bodies of T-11 and 12. Probe locates exact position for biopsy, and hollow-core sleeve is then slipped over probe to remove a section of bone and soft tissue for bacteriological and histological examination. Patient had an *S. aureus* infection.

misdiagnosed because of the similarity of these symptoms to those of other conditions.

In Rocco and Eyring's series, the sedimentation rate was increased above 22 mm/hour in 81 percent of the patients. This usually subsided to normal within 3 to 4 weeks. The white blood cell count was less than 8000/cu mm in 36 percent of the patients and above 11,000/cu mm in 43 percent. The differential cell count showed 70 percent polymorphonuclear cells in only 25 percent of patients.

The most common organism isolated in 9 of 23 direct cultures was *S. aureus*. Open biopsy was no more successful than needle biopsy for obtaining culture material. Of 6 cases tested, no positive blood culture was found. The most frequently used antibiotics were oxacillin, penicillin-G, and methicillin sodium.

Rocco and Eyring proposed that the hematogenous spread of the infectious agent stems from the fact that the embryonic disc has three major arterial supplies: periosteal vessels, axial vessels paralleling the notochord, and vessels descending from the central portion of the vertebral body. Disc space narrowing was explained by the possibility of water-binding capacity secondary to degradation of the protein polysaccharide complexes in the intercellular matrix;

the dense collagenous lamellae of the annulus fibrosus tend to confine the process within the disc space and inhibit extravertebral extension.

Spiegel and associates studied 48 children who had had disc space infections. These investigators concluded that: the condition is slightly more common in boys than in girls; there are no racial predilections; there seems to be no objective evidence that trauma is an etiological factor in the condition; and there is no evidence to suggest that the disease is related to avascular necrosis.

Radioisotope bone scanning may be extremely helpful in identifying pyogenic infections in the spine and sacroiliac joint. When a radioisotope such as 99-M technetium diphosphate is administered, increased activity can often be detected over the area of infection. This information, coupled with x-ray tomography, can aid early diagnosis and initiation of treatment in the adolescent.

Acute Direct Infection of The Spine

Occasionally, a patient develops a secondary infection after spinal puncture or surgical intervention. The infection generally is easily diagnosed since the patient is extremely irritable and has increased pain and all of the localized findings of an acute infectious process—such as a high sedimentation rate, temperature, and white blood cell count. The edges of the wound are often red and extremely tender, which indicates abscess formation.

Almost all spinal surgery results in a relatively large hematoma around the operative site, especially when spinal fusion has been performed. Since almost all surgical incisions are seeded with bacteria during surgery, most of these infections occur because of the excellent culture medium of the hematoma, or because too much dead space has been left in the wound and necrotic muscle and fascia are present.

When an acute infectious process of a postoperative wound is suspected, the patient should be taken immediately to the operating room and given a general inhalation anesthetic. The wound should then be properly prepped and draped, and all purulent material evacuated surgically. If a spinal fusion has been performed, the bone graft should not be removed; likewise, any inserted metal such as bone plates, wires, or distraction devices should be left in place. Irrigation tubes should be inserted and closed-suction irrigation promptly instituted using a rather rapid flow of saline through medium-sized irrigation tubes. The wound should be cultured and appropriate antibiotics started immediately. When cultures are available, antibiotics usually can be promptly changed and a specific antibiotic for the bacterium instituted.

Detergent solutions in the irrigation liquid sometimes provide mucolytic action in keeping the irrigation tubes free of necrotic plugs of muscle and fascia and keeping the suction tubes patent. The flow of the suction-irrigation system is reversed frequently, especially during the first 2 or 3 days, to keep the tubes from becoming plugged.

In addition to specific local antibiotics in the irrigation liquid, it is wise to give the patient systemic antibiotics for the same organism. A gram-negative antibiotic should be added to the irrigation system to keep it free of secondary invaders, which almost always are gram-negative organisms. The irrigation system should remain in place as long as possible, usually about 2 to 3 weeks. The skin edges then begin to leak, and the tubing must be removed. Systemic antibiotics should be continued for several months to prevent a recurrence of the infection.

The wound infection rate at our institution has dropped dramatically since we began a program of administering prophylactic antibiotics 1 day before spinal surgery, continuing antibiotics during surgery, and ending with 7 to 10 days of postoperative systemic antibiotics. In the last 580 major spinal operations, there has not been one gram-positive infection, and only two superficial gram-negative infections have been identified. This is in sharp contrast to wound infections and major septic complications encountered before we used prophylactic antbiotics.

Spinal Tuberculosis

Tuberculosis of the vertebral column is fortunately much less common now than in previous centuries. However, with the incidence of increasing drug and alcohol addiction in the adult population, more adolescents—especially in large cities—are being seen with spinal tuberculosis. Percival Pott was the first to describe spinal tuberculosis as a painful kyphotic deformity of the spine associated with paraplegia. The condition has since been referred to as Pott's disease. The spine is the most common site of skeletal tuberculosis, accounting for 50 percent of all cases. Any level of the spine can be involved, the lower thoracic region being the most common area, followed by the lumbar and upper thoracic regions.

Tuberculous infection of the spine usually begins in the cancellous bone of the vertebral body and only rarely in the posterior neural arch or transverse process. The area of infection slowly enlarges and eventually involves two or more adjacent vertebrae by extension beneath the anterior longitudinal ligament and directly across the intervertebral disc (Fig. 7-3). Occasionally, there can be multiple foci of involvement, with "skipped" areas of normal vertebrae in the spine and dissemination to distant vertebrae via connecting abscesses.

Because of the infectious process and the patient's immobility due to the disease, vertebral osteoporosis results. The vertebral bodies lose their strength and progressively collapse under the force of body weight. An angular kyphotic

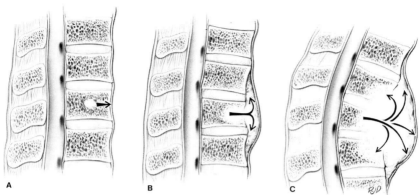

Fig. 7-3.   Localized spread of a tuberculosis infection. *A*. Infectious process begins in center of a vertebral body and points anteriorly to anterior longitudinal ligament. *B*. Anterior longitudinal ligament has been pushed away from vertebral body involved, and abscess extends to vertebral bodies above and below. *C*. Advanced abscess formation with erosion and destruction of all vertebral bodies involved. Because of loss of support, vertebral bodies then tend to collapse, causing a progressing kypohtic deformity that can lead to paralysis. (Redrawn after Tachdjian.)

deformity is therefore produced which, in its severe form, can lead to paraplegia. Kyphosis is most marked in the thoracic region because of the normal thoracic curve, and in some instances the patient's rib cage is actually supported by the pelvis on both sides.

Healing takes place slowly by gradual fibrosis and calcification of the tuberculous tissue. Eventually the fibrous tissue is ossified, and bony ankylosis of the collapsed vertebrae takes place. Occasionally, paravertebral abscesses form that resemble bird's nests (Fig. 7-4). These abscesses can gravitate along fascial planes and appear far from the original site, many times following the psoas sheath and pointing in the groin beneath the inguinal ligament.

The onset of tuberculous spondylitis is usually insidious, and the initial symptoms are vague, making the diagnosis difficult. A patient loses his appetite and then loses weight; he discontinues his usual activities such as sports and social functions. Almost all patients have increasing muscle spasm in the spine, which is quite obvious when they bend to pick up objects. If tuberculosis spondylitis is diagnosed promptly, chemotherapy can be instituted until the tuberculous focus is eradicated.

In the past, it was almost always taught that surgical decompression from the anterior or costotransverse route was essential to evacuate the abscess and

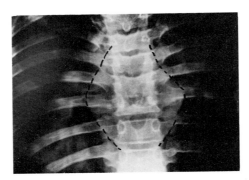

Fig. 7-4.   Bird's nest abscess in 12-year-old boy's thoracic spine. Disc space between 3 vertebrae in upper portion of abscess has collapsed. Lesion was biopsied, appropriate antituberculous therapy carried out, and total recovery obtained without surgical intervention.

cure the spondylitis. Spinal fusion at the time of decompression is most often advocated, especially by Hodgson and Stock in Hong Kong. Many of their patients had dramatic relief from the disease as well as from paraplegia by prompt anterior abscess evacuation and spinal fusion.

In this country, however, a chemotherapeutic approach has been applied during the past 20 years with relatively good success, especially when carried out over a long enough period. Friedman and Kapur have recently described the latest feeling in regard to chemotherapeutic treatment of tuberculosis. The "first line" antituberculosis drugs are considered to be rifampin, isoniazid, ethambutol, and streptomycin. The "second-line" antituberculosis drugs, which can be used in conjunction with the first four drugs mentioned, are ethionamide, para-aminosalicylic acid (PAS), cycloserine, pyrazinamide, capreomycin, viomycin, kanamycin, and amithiozone.

As current treatment, Friedman and Kapur recommend rifampin, isoniazid, and ethambutol for the first 6 months. At the end of 6 months, if the clinical and radiographic response is satisfactory, rifampin is discontinued and isoniazid and ethambutol are used in combination for the remaining 6 to 12 months.

Since many of these drugs have severe and frequent side effects, great caution must be used in prescribing them over long periods of time. Peripheral neuritis due to isoniazid can usually be prevented by the daily administration of vitamin B^6 (pyridoxine). Even when needle biopsy of a lesion suspected of being tuberculosis is negative for acid-fast bacilli, empirical treatment should be started. Under this modern chemotherapy, tuberculous lesions have been arrested and operative intervention prevented (Fig. 7-5 A, B). However, chemotherapy is expensive, especially when the patient is hospitalized. In this country, most surgical approaches are directed toward decompression for early

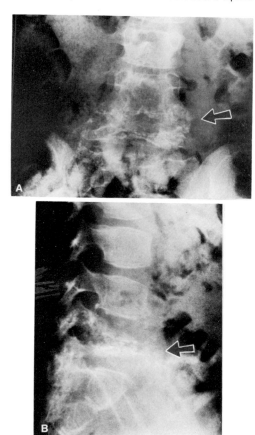

Fig. 7-5 *A,B.*   Severe tuberculous infection in 11-year-old-girl involves bodies of L-4 and 5. Films were taken 4 months after onset of symptoms and diagnosis. Patient was treated with antituberculous chemotherapy and later, lumbar spine fusion.

or late paraplegia. But chemotherapy is also used in conjunction with a surgical approach.

Brucellosis and fungal infections of the adolescent spine are fortunately quite uncommon. When they occur, they are treated in a similar manner as infections in the adult, usually with prolonged immobilization, bedrest, and surgical evacuation where indicated. In all forms of spinal infection, including tuberculosis, a long period of spinal immobilization is necessary in order to maintain the patient's spine in a proper alignment and allow spontaneous ankylosis to take place. If the immobilization is continued long enough, the spine remains stable and kyphotic deformity is prevented, thus averting the necessity for future reconstructive surgery to forestall progressive kyphosis.

REFERENCES

1. Ailshy RL, Staheli LT: Pyogenic infections of the sacroiliac joint in children. Radioisotope bone scanning as a diagnostic tool. Clin Orthop 100:96–100, 1974
2. Batson OV: The function of the vertebral veins and their role in the spread of metastases. Ann Surg 112:138, 1940
3. Bonfiglio M, Lange TA, Young MK: Pyogenic vertebral osteomyelitis. Clin Orthop 96:234–247, 1973
4. Craig, FS: Vertebral body biopsy. J Bone Joint Surg 38A:93, 1956
5. Friedman B: Chemotherapy of tuberculosis of the spine. J Bone Joint Surg 48A:451–474, 1966
6. Friedman B, Kapur VN: Newer knowledge of chemotherapy in the treatment of tuberculosis of bones and joints. Clin Orthop 97:5–15, 1973
7. Garcia A, Jr., Grantham SA: Hematogenous pyogenic vertebral osteomyelitis. J Bone Joint Surg 42A:429, 1960
8. Hibbs RA: An operation for progressive spinal deformities: a preliminary report of three cases from the service of the orthopaedic hospital. N Y Med J 93:1013–1016, 1911
9. Hodgson AR, Stock FE: Anterior spine fusion for the treatment of tuberculosis of the spine. J Bone Joint Surg 42A:295, 1960
10. Hodgson AR: Report on the findings and results in 300 cases of Pott's disease treated by anterior fusion of the spine. J West Pacific Orthop Asson 1:3–7, 1964
11. Kemp HBS, Jackson JW, Hall AJ, et al: Pyogenic infections occurring primarily in intervertebral discs. J Bone Joint Surg 55B:698–714, 1973
12. Menelaus, MB: Discitis: an inflammation affecting intervertebral discs in children. J Bone Joint Surg 46B:16, 1964
13. Nach CD, Keim HA: Prophylactic antibiotics in spine surgery. Ortho Rev II:6:27–30, 1973
14. Pott P: Remarks on that kind of palsy of the lower limbs which is frequently found to accompany a curvature of the spine and is supposed to be caused by it, in Medical Classics, vol 1. Baltimore, Williams & Wilkins, 1936, pp 271–322
15. Rocco HD, Eyring EJ: Intervertebral disc infections in children. Am J Dis Child
16. Spiegel PG, Kengla KW, Isaacson AS, et al: Intervertebral disc-space inflammation in children. J Bone Joint Surg 54A:284–296, 1972
17. Tachdjian MO: Pediatric Orthopaedics. Philadelphia, Saunders, 1972, Figs. 3–43, p 356

8
Scoliosis

Scoliosis is possibly the earliest evident affliction with which mankind was faced because it is such an obvious physical problem. Cave drawings from the Stone Age indicate that people had scoliosis and were aware of crude forms of treatment. For centuries man has been baffled by the etiology of scoliosis and its management.

Hippocrates was the first person to apply the term *scoliosis* to any curvature of the spine, and he originated early methods of treatment. Over 1000 years later, Paul of Aegina attempted to correct scoliosis gradually by binding the body to corrective splints. As early as 1582 Ambrose Paré instructed armorers in the development of iron corsets and cuirasses that were formed to the torsos of scoliosis patients in order to halt their deformity. During the Dark Ages, little was done to scoliosis, but toward the end of the 19th century, Hessing developed corsets to correct scoliotic deformities. In 1914 the first spine fusion for scoliosis was performed by Russell Hibbs at the old New York Orthapaedic Hospital. This first attempt at correcting scoliosis surgically attested to the fact that until that time no good brace or corset technique had been developed for the passive or active correction of scoliosis. It was not until 1946 that Blount and Schmidt of Milwaukee designed the Milwaukee brace, which has become a mainstay in the nonoperative treatment of scoliosis and kyphosis.

In recent years, the management of scoliosis with braces has been implemented with surgical instrumentation—namely, the Harrington system —which has revolutionized the surgical correction of these deformities. The Harrington technique is performed through the posterior approach to correct the curvature with a distraction and compression system, while autogenous bone is added to effect a spine fusion. This technique and efficient plaster immobilization methods aided by such developments as the Risser localizer cast and the Von Lackum surcingle cast technique, have allowed scoliotic patients early ambulation while maintaining excellent correction.

Recently, Dwyer of Australia devised an anterior approach to the thoracic and lumbar spine. He used a cable system threaded through vertebral screws to allow the correction of the curvature from the convex side. This technique has been especially helpful in treating patients for whom posterior surgery is too difficult or impossible because of infection or congenital defects of posterior elements, as in myelomeningocele.

The latest instrumentation to correct scoliosis has come from Bobechko, who attempted to insert electrodes on the convex side of the curve and direct electrical impulses to these from an external or internal source to allow "active" curve correction. The first such electrospinal instrumentation in the United States was performed at the New York Orthopaedic Hospital of the Columbia-Presbyterian Medical Center on May 1, 1975. This work is still in the experimental stage but shows promise for the future.

Although the management of the scoliotic pateint has changed many times during the last 60 years, we are still no closer to knowing the exact etiology of what is called "idiopathic" scoliosis. Therefore, treatment continues to consist of correcting the curvature after it develops, since no preventive form of treatment or definitive cure is yet known.

ETIOLOGY AND CLASSIFICATION

Despite extensive research on scoliosis and its causes, little is known about the etiology and pathogenesis of this condition. Cases of idiopathic scoliosis amount to approximately 80 percent of all spinal curvatures seen. Wynne-Davies in 1968 estimated the incidence of idiopathic scoliosis to be approximately 4 per 1000 for adolescent girls and about one-tenth this incidence for boys. In Minnesota, Kane and Moe found a prevalence rate of at least 1.33 per 1000 in 1970. In 1973 Brooks et al. reported a study of 841 adolescent school children with a scoliosis incidence of 11 percent verified on x-ray. Approximately 2 percent of the adult population has some form of scoliosis, but only in about 0.05 percent does this exceed 20°.

There are many theories on the etiology of scoliosis. In 1970 James pointed out that the only known cause of scoliosis is congenital malformation of the vertebrae. The cause of paralytic scoliosis with asymmetrical muscle paralysis is understood. However, the cause of idiopathic scoliosis is unknown, and thousands of various theories have been postulated, including growth disturbances of the vertebrae and apophyseal end plates, neuromuscular factors, gravitational forces, ligament defects, and hereditary, metabolic, chemical, and connective tissue factors.

Although all of these theories have been well researched, no specific cause for idiopathic scoliosis has been proven. Nevertheless the idiopathic group is being slowly whittled down as diagnostic techniques become more sophisticated and conditions that were originally thought to be "idiopathic" have been placed in a specific diagnostic category. Examples of this are the different forms of muscular atrophy and dystrophy.

However, the general group of idiopathic scoliosis remains, and evidence accumulated in recent years indicates that most of these cases are due to a genetic influence, possibly a dominant, sex-linked inheritance of a gene that has incomplete penetrance and variable expressivity. This means that the trait (but not the gene) can skip generations, and when expressed, the trait is manifested in different degrees of severity. For example, a mother or father may pass the gene to a daughter, but the child may have a milder or more severe curve than the parent and may even exhibit a different type of curve pattern altogether. Studies by MacEwen and Cowell in 1970 show that the sex linkage is to the X chromosome—that is, father to daughter or mother to son or daughter.

The author feels that idiopathic scoliosis usually is transmitted by one or both parents to their offspring. Therefore, the child receives a "dose" of scoliosis when the sperm and ovum combine. This is the same, in essence, as programming a computer to punch out a specific genetically coded message 12 or 13 years hence.

We all know people who have had pneumonia and some who have died of pneumonia. However, other people have pneumonia and barely lose a day's work. The reason why one person dies and the other is hardly affected is due to host resistance and the virulence of the organism involved.

Scoliosis can in many ways be compared to pneumonia. It is not an infectious process like pneumonia, but the genetic computer is set up when the zygote is formed. And a child will develop a specific curve of a certain degree that will be mild, moderate, or severe depending on the genetic dose imparted by the parent or parents at conception. If both parents had genetic factors from each of their family trees, then the child will probably receive a strong genetic dose of scoliosis and develop a severe curve.

In my practice, at least 40 percent of all children seen have a positive family history of scoliosis, and many children have brothers and sisters with the same condition. In fact, in two families 6 siblings are involved, and in one family 2 children required surgery and 3 wear braces for scoliosis (Fig. 8-1).

The genetic factors in idiopathic scoliosis seem so strong that I often advise young patients that there is a 30 to 40 percent chance that their offspring will develop scoliosis, especially if their children are girls. In addition, if that child marries a mate with scoliosis or a strong family history of scoliosis, a much higher incidence of scoliosis in their offspring can be expected.

Is it not strange that humans take such pride and caution in breeding family

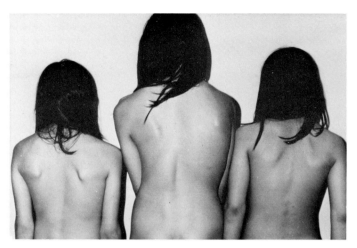

Fig. 8-1   3 sisters with idiopathic scoliosis. Girl in center required surgery, one on left was placed in a Milwaukee brace, and one on right was observed for future curve progression. A fourth sister, age 24, had a fairly fixed, 33° right thoracolumbar curve. Their mother and a maternal aunt had mild scoliosis.

pets and livestock, while they are almost lackadaisical when selecting a mate? We give almost no thought to pedigrees or the possibility of genetic deformities and malformations in offspring. We happily and carelessly start down the matrimonial road in symbiotic bliss without consideration of the fact that our choice of mate may well doom our children to serious medical problems and deformities.

The classification of spinal deformity has recently been modified by the Scoliosis Research Society and is shown in Table 8-I. Generally, scoliosis is classified as idiopathic, neuromuscular, or congenital. Years ago, paralytic scoliosis—especially that due to poliomyelitis—was the most common and most devastating form of scoliosis. With the advent of the Salk and Sabin vaccines, that paralytic form of scoliosis has been almost completely eradicated in this country and is being prevented in other countries throughout the world.

Idiopathic scoliosis seems to be slightly on the upswing, along with an increase in congenital anomalies, because many children who years ago would have died at birth or shortly thereafter are now living to adult life and developing progressive spinal deformities during their rapid growth years. Since it is impractical to discuss in detail in this text all of the possible etiologies of scoliosis, only the major theories according to the classification in Table 8-1 will be discussed in order.

Table 8-1
Classification of Spine Deformity

I. Idiopathic
  A. Infantile: 0–3 years
    1. Resolving
    2. Progressive
  B. Juvenile: 4–puberty onset
  C. Adolescent: Puberty +
  D. Adult: females, (18+), males, (20+)
II. Neuromuscular
  A. Neuropathic
    1. Upper motor neuron lesion
      a. Cerebral palsy
      b. Spinocerebellar degeneration
        i. Friedreich's
        ii. Charcot-Marie-Tooth
        iii. Roussy-Lévy
      c. Syringomyelia
      d. Spinal cord tumor
      e. Spinal cord trauma
      f. Other
    2. Lower motor neuron lesion
      a. Poliomyelitis
      b. Other viral myelitides
      c. Traumatic
      d. Spinal muscular atrophy
        i. Werdnig-Hoffmann
        ii. Kugelberg-Welander
      e. Myelomeningocele (paralytic)
    3. Dysautonomia (Riley-Day)
    4. Other
  B. Myopathic
    1. Arthrogryposis
    2. Muscular dystrophy
      a. Duchenne (pseudohypertrophic)
      b. Limb-girdle
      c. Facioscapulohumeral
    3. Fiber-type disproportion
    4. Congenital hypotonia
    5. Myotonia dystrophica
    6. Other
III. Congenital
  A. Congenital scoliosis
    1. Failure of formation
      a. Wedge

        b.   Hemivertebra
    2. Failure of segmentation
        a.   Unilateral bar
        b.   Bilateral (''fusion'')
    3. Mixed
  B.   Congenital kyphosis
    1. Failure of formation
    2. Failure of segmentation
    3. Mixed
  C.   Congenital lordosis
  D.   Associated with neural tissue defect
    1. Myelomeningocele
    2. Meningocele
    3. Spinal dysraphism
        a.   Diastematomyelia
        b.   Other
IV.   Neurofibromatosis
V.   Mesenchymal
  A.   Marfan's syndrome
  B.   Homocystinuria
  C.   Ehlers-Danlos syndrome
  D.   Other
VI.   Traumatic
  A.   Fracture or dislocation (nonparalytic)
  B.   Postirradiation
  C   Postlaminectomy
  D.   Other
VII. Soft tissue contractures
  A.   Postempyema
  B.   Burns
  C.   Other
VIII. Osteochondrodystrophies
  A.   Achondroplasia
  B.   Spondyloepiphyseal dysplasia
  C.   Diastrophic dwarfism
  D.   Mucopolysaccharidoses
IX.   Scheuermann's disease
X.   Infection
  A.   Tuberculosis
  B.   Bacterial
  C.   Fungal
  D.   Parasitic
  E.   Other
XI.   Tumor
  A.   Benign

B.   Malignant
XII.   Rheumatoid disease
   A.   Juvenile rheumatoid
   B.   Adult rheumatoid
   C.   Marie-Strümpel
XIII. Metabolic
   A.   Rickets
   B.   Juvenile osteoporosis
   C.   Osteogenesis imperfecta
XIV. Related to lumbosacral area
   A.   Spondylolisthesis
   B.   Spondylolysis
   C.   Other congenital anomalies
   D.   Other
XV.   Thoracogenic
   A.   Post-thoracoplasty
   B.   Post-thoracotomy
   C.   Other
XVI. Hysterical
XVII. Functional
   A.   Postural
   B.   Secondary to short leg
   C.   Other

PATHOMECHANICS OF SCOLIOSIS

Scoliosis is an extremely complex condition because it involves not only a lateral bend in the spine, but also consists of a rotational deformity of the vertebral column around its longitudinal axis. Because of this rotation, the ribs in the thoracic region follow the torque imposed on them by the twisting spinal column and become most prominent on the convex side (Fig. 8-2A). The ribs push the scapulae backward and cause an unsightly rib deformity; in many instances they cause the spine to go out of balance. That is, the head does not remain centered over the pelvis, but the head and upper torso fall to the right or left of the gluteal cleft, causing altered spinal mechanics and subsequent degenerative joint disease in adult life. As vertebral rotation continues, the spinous processes of the vertebrae involved in the major curve rotate toward the concavity of the curve. The ribs on the concavity become crowded together and are carried forward so that there is usually an anterior prominence of the ribs on the concave side. The ribs on the convexity push the scapula backward to cause the usual "winging."

In the initial stages, mild scoliosis can be considered functional—i.e., it is

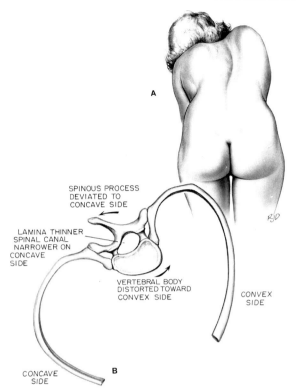

SPINOUS PROCESS
DEVIATED TO
CONCAVE SIDE

LAMINA THINNER
SPINAL CANAL
NARROWER ON
CONCAVE
SIDE

VERTEBRAL BODY
DISTORTED TOWARD
CONVEX SIDE

CONVEX
SIDE

CONCAVE   B
SIDE

Fig. 8-2.*A* View from behind, patient with advanced right
thoracic scoliosis. Thoracic cage is asymmetric and rotational deformity of ribs on convex side pushes back scapula. *B*. Cross-
section of thoracic vertebra seen from below. Convex side changes
consist of vertebral body distorted toward that side, thickened
lamina, and wide pedicle. On concave side, spinal canal is ovoid
and distorted toward that side, pedicle is thin and wafer-shaped, and
lamina is also thin. Spinous process is usually deviated to concave
side.

not structural and can easily be corrected by side bending. After a curve has
been present for a long time, it developes a structural component and cannot be
corrected by side bending. A fixed, or structural, deformity is therefore present
which must be corrected by some type of external or internal device. Lateral
curvature and rotation occur in unison to continue the deformity, especially
during periods of rapid growth.

As the vertebrae rotate, the disc spaces become narrowed on the concave
side and widened on the convex side of the curve. The vertebral bodies become
wedged and the laminae become thicker on the convex side, along with

thickening of the pedicles on the same side. On the concave side in the thoracic spine, the pedicles become thin and waferlike with an ovoid configuration of the spinal canal, with narrowing on the concave side. The vertebral body is distorted toward the convex side, and the spinous process is deviated to the concave side (Fig. 8-2B).

IDIOPATHIC SCOLIOSIS

For years scoliosis with no known cause was referred to as idiopathic. As mentioned before, there is now evidence that most idiopathic scoliosis is genetic. Idiopathic scoliosis occurs about six times more frequently in adolescent girls than in boys and accounts for approximately 70 percent of all cases of scoliosis. The etiology of idiopathic scoliosis has previously been mentioned; however, Zorab in 1968 pointed out that there are basically four possible groups of causes for structural idiopathic scoliosis. He felt the cause may lie in the bony vertebral column and adjacent ribs; in the surrounding muscles, nerves, or blood supply; in an inequality of growth rates of the two sides of the body; or, finally, in the connective tissue.

Connective tissue metabolism in patients with idiopathic scoliosis has been investigated for many years in an attempt to discover any disorder. In 1968 Ponseti found an excess total hexosamine content in iliac crest biopsies of patients with idiopathic adolescent scoliosis. He concluded that excess hexosamine was also produced in cartilage cells of the vertebral growth plates and their intervertebral discs. Ponseti also found evidence of decreased collagen formation in the intervertebral discs, which he felt led to the rotation that occurs, especially in the thoracic and lumbar spine.

Rats fed on a diet of β-aminopropionitrile have defective collagen formation and develop lathryism and scoliosis. A high α-β chain ratio in skin samples from patients with Marfan's syndrome and from patients with homocysteinuria suggests defective collagen formation in both syndromes. It has been suggested that homocysteine may limit collagen cross-linkage. In both of these conditions, scoliosis is a frequent problem.

It has recently been observed that although scoliosis has been broken down into infantile, juvenile, and adolescent groups, there probably are few patients with true adolescent scoliosis. Most of these children have a mild curve when they are juveniles, but the curve does not really express itself until the rapid growth spurt of adolescence.

Of 725 patients with idiopathic scoliosis studied at the duPont Institute in Delaware, 111 had positive family histories. Of the next 100 patients examined with scoliotic curves over 10°, 10 percent of their siblings also had scoliosis over 10°. In a recent school screening in Delaware, 315,000 patients were examined between September 1962 and June 1972. Of these patients, 1461 were referred for further investigation of spinal anomalies or other orthopedic disorders, especially in the lower extremities. School screening is an extremely effective means of detecting scoliosis in its early stages, and nationwide screening efforts are being instituted since the earlier a curve is detected the more promptly appropriate treatment and referral to proper facilities can be instituted.

Infantile Idiopathic Scoliosis

The infantile idiopathic scoliosis group consists of those between birth and 3 years of age. Generally, scoliosis in this age range is noted during the first year of life. It is much more common in England and usually occurs in males; most of these young boys have a left thoracic curve. The majority of these cases resolve spontaneously, even if untreated. However, some patients develop extremely rigid structural curves and marked deformities if left alone.

Juvenile Idiopathic Scoliosis.

The juvenile age group includes children between the age of 4 and the onset of puberty. Juvenile idiopathic scoliosis affects both sexes equally. Most of the children have right thoracic or double major curves, and many of these resolve spontaneously but must be observed closely, since some do get progressively worse and require treatment.

Adolescent Idiopathic Scoliosis.

Adolescent idiopathic scoliosis is diagnosed when the curve is noted between the onset of puberty and skeletal maturity. These curves are probably present during the juvenile years (equally in boys and girls), but for some reason girls tend to have progressive curves as they reach adolescence. Adolescent idiopathic curves may or may not progress during growth. Usually the younger the child when the structural curve develops, the more serious is the prognosis. Most of these structural curves have to progress rapidly, especially during the adolescent growth spurt, whereas small nonstructural curves may remain flexible for long periods and never require treatment.

A curve that does not correct on a recumbent side-bending x-ray is a structural curve (which almost always progresses Fig. 8-3). The term "major" is used to designate the larger curve, and this is almost always structural. A "minor" curve is usually a compensatory curve, is smaller than the major curve, and can also be structural. It is better not to call the major curve primary since this implies a temporal relationship, and in most scoliosis patients it is difficult to determine which curve appeared first.

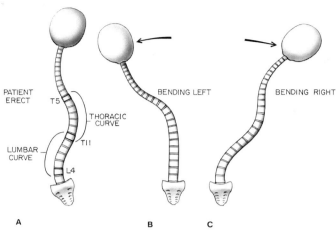

Fig. 8-3   Side-bending to determine whether a curve is structural or nonstructural. *A*.
Patient is erect and both curves seem to be in balance. *B*. Patient bends to left and lumbar
curve straightens and overcorrects, indicating a functional and nonstructural curve. If
surgery were required for upper curve, this curve would not need to be fused. *C*. The
patient bends to right side and upper curve does not correct completely, indicating that
thoracic curve is structural and requires treatment. All vertebrae in a structural curve
plus 1 vertebra above and 2 below the curve should be included in the fusion area. If on
side-bending a compensatory curve is found to be nonstructural, it need not be included
in the fusion site.

Curve Patterns

Curve patterns in idiopathic scoliosis generally fit into one of five distinctive types. The first and perhaps the most common, curve pattern is the double
major curve. There are two curves of great prominence, both which are
structural and usually of the same magnitude. Double major curves can be right
thoracic and left lumbar, which is the most frequent combination, or they can
both be located in the thoracic region, with a right thoracic-left thoracic curve,
or a right thoracic–left thoracolumbar curve. Sometimes there is a left
thoracolumbar with a right low lumbar curve, and occasionally all these curve
patterns are reversed.

Often an adolescent girl with a strong propensity for scoliosis develops a
right thoracic curve. In an effort to right itself, the spine develops compensatory
curves above and below this thoracic curve. The patient therefore must have
three separate curves, with a cervical curve to the left and a lumbar curve to the
left to try to keep the head balanced over the pelvis and compensate for the right
thoracic curve. A major right thoracic curve combined with a minimal left
lumbar curve is sometimes referred to as an intermediate curve pattern.

As the patient grows, the lumbar curve often increases and becomes more rigid, changing from a nonstructural to a structural curve. If the lumbar curve increases in magnitude to the size of the thoracic curve, the pattern has then changed to a double major pattern, with the typical right thoracic–left lumbar combination. In most cases the thoracic curve runs from T-5 to T-11 or 12, and the left lumbar curve runs from T-11 or 12 to L-4 or 5.

Because these curves are symmetrical and well balanced, they are less deforming than single curves, but severe progression of double major curves leads to a short trunk, and these patients appear "stunted" (Fig. 8-4C). For this reason, when double major curves become excessive, they require treatment, especially if the lumbar curve causes a severe rotational deformity with subsequent degenerative changes and pain.

Thoracic curves are the second most common idiopathic pattern, with the end vertebrae at T-4, 5, or 6 at the upper limit and T-11, 12, or L-1 as the lower limit (Fig. 8-4A). These curves are usually highly structural (they do not correct on side bending. Because of the severe vertebral rotation, the ribs on the convex side become badly deformed, causing a cosmetic problem and seriously impairing cardiopulmonary function, especially when curves exceed 60°. Thoracic curves are most often to the right and can achieve severely extreme proportions, in many instances becoming as great as 150° to 180° (Fig. 8-5A, B).

The thoracolumbar curve, a fairly common idiopathic curve pattern, usually consists of both right and left types. The upper end vertebra is T-4, 5, or 6, and the lower end vertebra is L-2, 3, or 4. In addition, if there is a right thoracolumbar curve, there is usually a compensatory upper left thoracic or cervical curve and a lower left lumbar curve. Thoracolumbar curves are usually less deforming than thoracic curves; however, because they are long curves and involve the lumbar spine, thoracolumbar curves can cause the spine to go markedly "out of balance" and lead to severe degenerative changes in later life. They should therefore be promptly and aggressively treated when first detected. These curves probably have the greatest propensity to continue to get worse during adult life (Fig. 8-4B).

Lumbar curves are fairly common and usually run from T-11 or 12 to L-5. They are generally to the left in 65 percent of cases. The thoracic spine above usually does not develop a structural compensatory curve, but remains flexible to keep the spine in balance. These curves are not very deforming cosmetically, but because of the rotation that occurs in a lumbar curve, they do lead to severe degenerative arthritic changes in later life and cause increased lumbar pain, especially associated with pregnancy and thereafter. They also tend to become more severe long after full maturity and many continue to do so throughout adult life (Fig 8-4D).

The fifth group of idiopathic curves includes cervicothoracic curves, which are uncommon and generally go to the left and run from C-4 or 5 to T-4

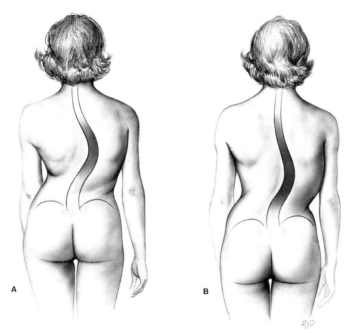

Fig. 8-4. Curve patterns in idiopathic scoliosis. *A*. Right thoracic scoliosis with marked asymmetry of thoracic cage. *B*. Thoracolumbar scoliosis; curves tend to be out of balance, with head displaced away from midline of pelvis. *C*. Double major idiopathic scoliosis showing right thoracic–left lumbar curve pattern, the most common double major pattern. *D*. Lumbar scoliosis, which is most commonly to left. Pelvic obliquity is marked on concave side, which leads to apparent leg length discrepancy.

or 5. They rarely cause pain but distort the shoulders and clavicles causing a cosmetic problem.

The deformity is variable depending on how many ribs are involved. Severe forms are difficult to treat because adequate purchase on the scapulae and upper thoracic ribs is hard to achieve through bracing or other nonoperative means due to the presence of the upper extremity.

Because idiopathic scoliosis arises in an apparently healthy child and does not generally cause any pain, the condition is rarely detected during the early stages. Affected children often are also missed in routine pediatric examinations or camp physicals; because they are in good health, their spines are rarely examined. Also, many curves begin insidiously and progress in a short time. Some curves have been observed to progress 40° over a 3-month period, leading to an extremely severe deformity that the parents had hardly recognized several months before. Most of these curves are detected by a dance instructor or by a mother who is sewing a dress for her daughter and finds that a hemline is

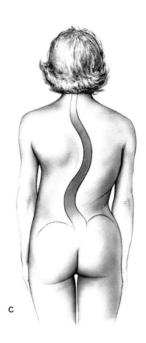
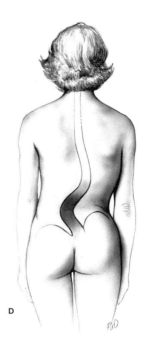

C   D

too long on one side. The deformity may be noted when the patient is in a
bathing suit while the family is on vacation.

Unfortunately, parents usually feel guilty about the scoliotic deformity,
especially when they find out that in most cases it is genetic. They berate
themselves for transmitting it to their child and for not having detected the
condition earlier. They often are angry that their physician did not notice the
condition during routine physicals. Hair styles, especially in girls, many times
cover up most of the spine. Most young girls are so modest about their dressing
habits that the curves tend to become quite advanced before they are detected.

When the family is first seen in the orthopedist's office, they must be
assured that everything will be done to treat their child. They must be told that
they have not been negligent parents, and that they should not blame a family
member with scoliosis for transmitting the condition to their child. After
examining the child, the physician should examine all siblings and instruct the
family to notify all relatives that they should have their children examined
because of the strong genetic propensity for scoliosis.

Many unanswered questions about idiopathic scoliosis are being carefully
studied by the Scoliosis Research Society. First, why do perfectly healthy
adolescent girls develop such severe spinal deformities? Why is it a 50 percent

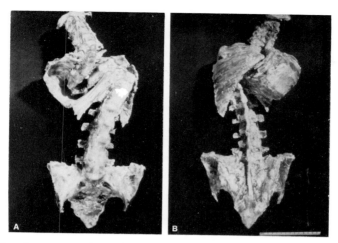

Fig. 8-5. Autopsy specimen from adult who died of cardiopulmonary problems associated with scoliosis. During early adolescence this woman's spine was straight. Scoliosis does progress in many adults. (Courtesy James J. Hamilton, M.D)

female condition at age 10 but an 80 percent female condition at 14? Why are double major curves almost always right thoracic and left lumbar? Why aren't thoracic curves in adolescents left sided? Why do infants with the condition have left-sided thoracic curves, and why are most of these males? Why do 90 percent of infantile curves resolve before age 3, but after that age why do 98 percent of them get worse? Why do 80 percent of 12-year-old girls with small curves have small curves at age 15, while 20 percent become drrastically worse? And why do two children of the same age, sex, and curve type respond so differently to brace treatment—one ending up with a beautifully straight spine and the other getting progressively worse, eventually needing surgery? Can all of these questions be answered by the "genetic dosage" of scoliosis a child receives at conception?

Adult Scoliosis

Many cases of scoliosis do not stop progressing when the patient has reached full maturity. For years it was thought that when the iliac epiphysis was completely closed and all other forms of maturation were complete, scoliotic curves would never progress. Nothing could be further from the truth! Old axioms and cliches die a slow death, especially if untrue. In scoliosis clinics throughout the world, patients with significant curves at full maturity have developed severe debilitating and progressive curves in later adult life. This is especially true in female scoliotics after pregnancies.

Scoliosis that exceeds 60° by the Cobb method causes progressive cardiac and pulmonary disturbances in later life. These changes often lead to cor pulmonale and early death. Most of these patients are not seen by an average orthopedic surgeon but come to the attention of the pulmonary physiologist and scoliosis specialist after they have started to die. Several investigators have studied the prognosis for patients with untreated idiopathic scoliosis. In 1968 Nachemson reported a 35-year follow-up study on 117 scoliosis patients. He found that nearly half had some form of cardiopulmonary trouble. There was an increase of over 100 percent in mortality of these patients when compared with the general population. In advanced curves, the mortality was four times greater. Nilsonne and Lundgren also reported the same results in a 50-year follow-up of 100 patients. They showed that a significant number of female patients never married.

Collis and Ponseti followed 195 scoliosis patients for an average of 24 years and showed that the decrease in vital capacity was proportional to their degree of scoliosis. In my practice, many adult patients tell me that they had rather minimal or moderate curves at age 21. They all admit that during pregnancy and with increasing age the curvature has increased; when they are seen, many of these patients have curves above the 50° or 60° range (Cobb).

These patients are hard to mollify since many feel that they have had improper medical advice and poor management in the past. Many physicians that they have visited have told them not to worry about their problem and that their curves would never get worse. This is totally untrue—*scoliosis often progresses in adults*, (Fig. 8-5), especially if the curves are out of balance.

It is generally felt that scoliosis curves in adults progress 1° per year of adult life, and generally 6° to 8° with each pregnancy. The same hormones that circulate throughout the body to allow softening of the pelvic ligaments and the birth of a child also seem to affect the ligaments of the thoracic and lumbar spine. (The main hormone is thought to be *relaxin*.) In some patients, as much as 30° of progression has been noted with one or two pregnancies. *The feeling among physicians that scoliosis will not progress in the adult is unfounded and untrue.* (Figure 8-6.)

All scoliotic patients should be observed regularly throughout their lives and not only until maturity. Many times the "watch and wait" attitude merely makes the patient feel complacent and people drift away from medical care until their deformity becomes so severe that they return for treatment when it is extremely difficult to administer and the rigid curves are almost impossible to correct. The indications for surgical treatment in the adult are pain, increasing deformity, decreasing pulmonary capacity, neurological impairment, and progressive cosmetic deformity.

We do not know why scoliosis progresses in adults, except that connective tissues do change with the age of the patient. This "aging" seems to depend on the number of cross-linkages between collagen molecules. The progression of

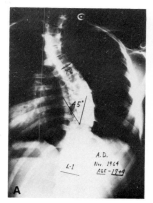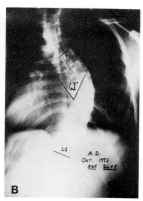

Fig. 8-6. Scoliosis progression in mature patient. *A*. At age 17 years and 9 months, patient had a 45° right thoracic curve. Several orthopedic surgeons advised against treatment because they were certain curve would never get worse. *B*. At age 26 and 8 months, thoracic curve has increased to 61°. Symptoms increased markedly and included pain and moderate shortness of breath. Surgery was carried out with a good result.

scoliosis is closely connected with spinal growth, and adolescent idiopathic scoliotic girls are taller than normal girls.

In 1968 Ponseti suggested that idiopathic scoliosis be called "discogenic" scoliosis. He found a severe derangement in the mucopolysaccharides of the intervertebral discs of girls with idiopathic scoliosis. Increasing curves in the adult spine seem to result as an increase in wedging in the intervertebral soft parts, especially in the disc. This has been proven by x-ray techniques that show compression of the intervertebral discs on the concave side and widening of the discs on the convex side, but no changes directly in the structure of the bodies of the vertebrae.

The fact that certain scoliotic patients continue to get worse in adult life merely indicates that these patients probably have inherited a greater degree of scoliosis from their parents than others, and this genetic pattern tends to continue throughout their adult life. The best treatment for a scoliosis patient is prompt referral to a physician or clinic handling a large volume of these cases. People at these centers are best equipped to handle scoliotic patients and halt the curves before they assume drastic proportions. The worst thing to do for a patient is to tell her not to worry about the condition or to just observe her and watch the curve progress.

Progressing scoliosis in a young person causes great mental and physical anguish. Who knows how many feelings have been hurt because of unkind remarks, how many jobs have been lost because of physical deformity, and how

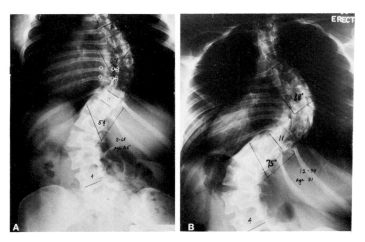

Fig. 8-7 *A*.   25-year-old woman with right thoracic curve of 62° and left lumbar curve of 54°. Scoliosis surgery had been advised when she was a teenager, but her family refused treatment. She also had asymptomatic grade II spondylolisthesis of L 5. By age 25 curves had increased, and she had 2 children within 3 years. *B*. At age 31; increase from 62° to 88° in thoracic curve and from 54° to 75° in lumbar curve. Spondylolisthesis at L-5 had increased to grade III.

much loss of self-image has been suffered by the scoliosis patient as she moves from budding adolescence into adult ugliness while watching her body grow increasingly deformed (Fig. 8-7A, B).

In America we spend much time and money correcting crooked teeth with proper orthodontic care, but many times we neglect a spinal deformity that is much more important both physiologically and emotionally. We must strive for better school screening methods, more physician and nurse education, and increased public awareness that scoliosis can be well controlled with prompt recognition and treatment.

NEUROMUSCULAR SCOLIOSIS

Neuromuscular scoliosis accounts for a small segment of the total number of spinal curvatures seen. Although the incidence of neuromuscular scoliosis is low, the frequency of scoliosis curves in neuromuscular disease is extremely high. Several factors separate neuromuscular from idiopathic scoliosis. First, the cause of neuromuscular scoliosis is known. In idiopathic scoliosis the curve may progress, but in neuromuscular scoliosis both the curve *and* the disease may progress. Second, with neuromuscular disease, the curves appear earlier in

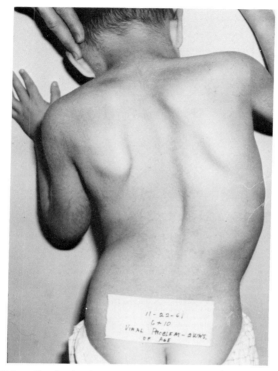

Fig. 8-8.   Cerebral palsy scoliosis due to viral infection first detected at 2 weeks of age. Patient had rigid progressing curve that
was held for several years in a Milwaukee brace and eventually
fused.

life progress rapidly, and almost always continue to progress throughout adult
life. Quite commonly, patients with neuromuscular scoliosis die of pulmonary
causes combined with progression of neuromuscular disease.

Neuromuscular scoliosis is classified as neuropathic or myopathic (Table
8-1). Neuropathic types include upper motor neuron lesions—cerebral palsy,
spinocerebellar degeneration, syringomyelia, spinal cord tumors, and spinal
cord trauma (Fig. 8-8 and 8-9). In almost all of these diseases, a muscular
imbalance on one side of the spine causes an overpull of the stronger muscles
leading to progressing deformity.

Sometimes the condition is correctable by surgical or x-ray treatment, as
in the case of spinal cord tumors (Fig. 8-10). However, the condition often is
neurologically progressive, as in syringomyelia. In recent years we have found
that many of these patients continue to live long beyond the usual life span of a

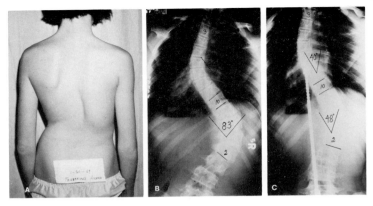

Fig. 8-9. 14-year-old girl with Friedreich's ataxia and progressing right thoracolumbar scoliosis of 83°. Surgery corrected major curve to 48°. Neurological condition progressed slowly over next 6 years, and in spite of poor prognosis, she has been leading a relatively enjoyable life.

particular disease. Because of this, these patients should be aggressively treated when first seen, either by bracing or surgical means, to allow them to have as normal and long a functional life as possible.

Neuropathic Scoliosis

The neuropathic lower motor neuron lesions include poliomyelitis, other viral myelitides, traumatic injuries to the lower motor neurons, spinal muscular atrophy, and myelomeningocele (Figs. 8-11, 8-12, and 8-13). As previously

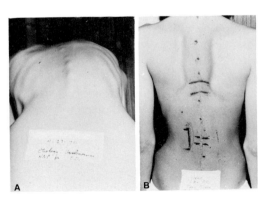

Fig. 8-10. 12-year-old girl first seen with right thoracolumbar scoliosis and severe pain. Herniated disc or osteoid osteoma was suspected until further evaluation, including a myelogram, revealed a spinal cord tumor. B. After irradiation, scoliosis is almost completely resolved.

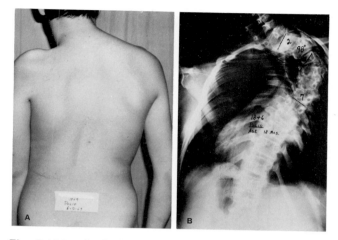

Fig. 8-11*A*.   Scoliosis secondary to poliomyelitis at age 18 months. Patient had high thoracic scoliosis with progressing curvature leading to partial paraplegia at age 18 years and 7 months. *B*. Patient was then admitted for halofemoral traction and spinal fusion in situ, with complete resolution of neurological symptoms.

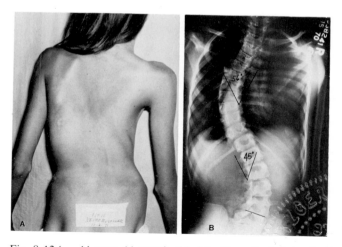

Fig. 8-12*A*.   11-year, 11-month-old girl with scoliosis secondary to smallpox reaction at 6 months of age. She developed neuromuscular scoliosis consisting of left thoracic–right lumbar curves. Whenever a left thoracic curve pattern is noted in a scoliotic patient always consider some other type of etiology since this curve pattern is highly uncommon in "idiopathic" curves.

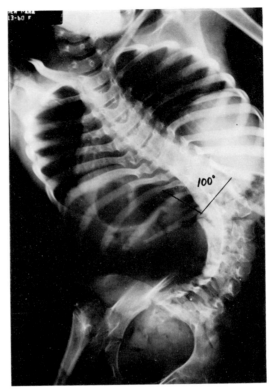

Fig. 8-13. Severe right thoracolumbar scoliosis secondary to blood transfusion reaction at birth. Spinal fusion was attempted repeatedly, but multiple pseudarthroses are still present, with increase in curve.

mentioned, poliomyelitis used to be the most common cause of scoliosis because it was such a common disease until preventive vaccines were developed. Now, however, myelomeningocele is the major lower motor neuron lesion resulting in paralytic scoliosis (Fig. 8-14).

As in most forms of neuromuscular scoliosis, the myelomeningocele patient develops a long, C-shaped curve that generally extends from the occiput to the sacrum. The degree of the curve is directly proportional to the severity of the myelomeningocele. Children whose posterior elements are completely open for a long section of the spine and who have a severe paralytic disorder often have extremely severe curves that are almost impossible to hold by either conservative or surgical means. If the patient has an extremely low IQ and will not be a functional member of society, it is probably best to defer treatment and

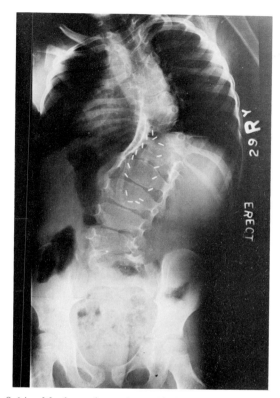

Fig. 8-14. Myelomeningocele scoliosis in patient with diastematomyelia at T-12 and L-1. Neurosurgical clips outline area of
diastematomyelia. All foot problems were relieved after intraspinal
surgery, and eventually anterior spinal fusion was successful.

allow the condition to follow its natural course. However, some of these
patients are quite bright and all attempts at spinal correction and stabilization
should be made.

During the early years of life when the patient's spine is quite flexible, a
corrective corset can usually exert proper pressure to allow the spine to grow as
straight as possible. However, during adolescence surgical means of correction
is usually necessary and these techniques are often difficult because there are no
posterior elements to which to attempt a spinal fusion. In addition, the iliac
crests and pelvis are usually hypoplastic and do not provide good sources for
graft material to effect a fusion. With the advent of Dwyer's anterior technique,
more of these patients are surgically correctable; however, the poor quality of
their bone substance still makes them extremely difficult to treat surgically.

Familial dysautonomia (Riley-Day syndrome) is a hereditary neuropathic disease due to an autosomal recessive gene occurring mainly in children who are Ashkenazi Jews. The disorder affects small, unmyelinated autonomic nerve fibers, causing a severe muscle imbalance leading to marked scoliosis and kyphosis. The patients are extremely high surgical risks because of cardiovascular system instability and chronic lung disease.

Neuromuscular-Myopathic Scoliosis

The second type of neuromuscular scoliosis is myopathic scoliosis, which includes arthrogryposis, muscular dystrophy, fiber-type disproportion, congenital hypotonia, and myotonia dystrophica. Arthrogryposis, also known as amyoplasia congenita, is a disorder causing extremely rigid and deformed joints in the newborn infant. The affected joints may be held in a position of flexion or extension, in a rigid path of movement (Fig. 8-15). Some investigators feel that the primary site of involvement is in the muscles, whereas others contend that the primary abnormality consists of an absence or agenesis of anterior horn cells in the spinal cord similar to that seen in Werdnig-Hoffmann disease, with secondary denervation atrophy in muscle. These children many times develop severe scoliosis that is difficult to correct by either surgical or nonoperative means.

Scoliosis also develops in the muscular dystrophies, which can be the pseudohypertrophic type of Duchenne, limb-girdle, or facioscapulohumeral

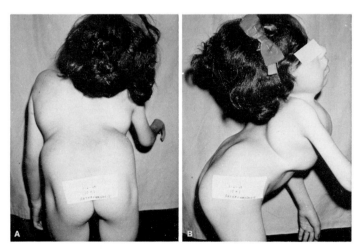

Fig. 8-15.   10-year, 1-month-old girl with severe arthrogryposis and fixed deformities that were not amenable to any type of surgical or brace treatment.

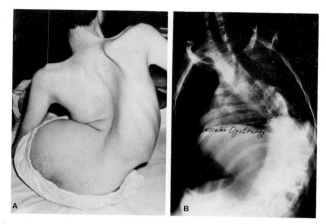

Fig. 8-16. Severe muscular dystrophy in a 16-year-old boy with a 140° right thoracolumbar curve. His respiratory reserve was so poor that attempts at correction were confined to nonoperative care using a polypropylene corset.

type. In all types of muscular dystrophy, the amount of deformity depends on how severely affected the patient is. Long C-shaped curves develop and are usually best treated by bracing or maintenance with a molded corset (Fig. 8-16). However, some of these people do live well beyond the twenties and thirties, and if their prognosis seems favorable for a reasonably prolonged life, surgical intervention can be helpful.

The other types of myopathic neuromuscular scoliosis basically require the same forms of treatment as those mentioned above. Again treatment depends on the severity of the condition and the patient's spinal instability. Even though most of these patients are wheelchair bound, a stable spine helps them maintain their balance and operate their chairs more efficiently.

CONGENITAL SCOLIOSIS

Congenital scoliosis was mentioned in Chapter 1 (Fig. 1-4). It can consist of failure of (1) formation or (2) segmentation. The former can be partial or complete and unilateral or bilateral. Partial failure of formation that is unilateral results in wedged vertebrae, whereas failure of formation that is complete and unilateral results in hemivertebrae. Failure of segmentation can be unilateral or bilateral, and unilateral failure leads to unsegmented bars of bone that act as a tethering mechanism, causing the opposite side to grow at a disproportionate rate and leading to severe scoliotic deformities. Bilateral failure of segmentation causes block vertebrae and this leads to a shortness in total trunk height (Fig. 1-4).

Hemivertebrae tend to cause increasing scoliotic curves because the propensity for growth of that center of ossification in the hemivertebrae leads the spine to tilt in the opposite direction. When a hemivertebra on one side is combined with unilateral bars on the opposite side, spinal deformities can be severe.

Investigators have previously stated incorrectly that congenital scoliosis is not progressive. Only about 25 percent of congenital scoliosis does not progress; of the 75 percent of patients in whom the condition does progress, about half develop extremely severe deformities generally requiring a combination of surgery and bracing (Fig. 8-17).

Because of the nature of congenital scoliosis, we many times see mixed deformities consisting of unilateral bars, hemivertebrae, and fused ribs (Fig. 4-1). These deformities tend to become rigid, and the lack of flexibility and correctability requires extremely prompt recognition and treatment. The physician must determine which curvatures are likely to progress and which ones are not, and also which curvatures will continue to a severe deformity and at what rate. Factors to be considered in evaluating congenital scoliosis are the magnitude of curve, the years of skeletal spinal growth remaining, the specific nature and type of anomaly present, and the area of the spine in which the anomaly is located. For years students were taught that spinal surgery should not be performed until the spine is fully mature. This is a complete fallacy,

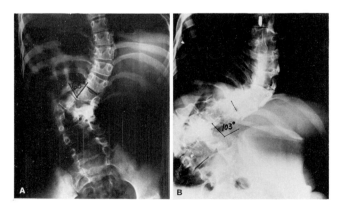

Fig. 8-17A.   11-year-old girl with 60° congenital scoliosis due to unilateral bars on concave side and hemivertebrae on convex side. Surgery was strongly advised at that time, but family refused. B. Same patient 5 years later with severe curve increase to 103°. Right iliac crest is practically touching spinal column, and patient is paraplegic.

since a short, straight spine is much better than a short, crooked spine. As soon as a congenital curve is noted to progress, it should be treated aggressively with a surgical approach consisting of spinal fusion in situ. Nevertheless, even after surgical correction by spine fusion, most of these patients require Milwaukee bracing until they are totally mature because the living spine continues to be governed by Wolff's law (living bone responds to stresses placed on it).

In addition, many patients with congenital scoliosis and kyphosis require multiple operative procedures staged over their entire growth period, and these must be combined with bracing or cast correction during the intervening years. Congenital curves tend to progress insidiously, and unless serial x-rays of the child are compared with the original x-rays, the curves can continue to progress at an unrelenting pace. Since these curves are so rigid structurally, they are generally impossible to correct once the curve is severe. Therefore, a congenital fusion or an operative fusion must be closely watched and often protected by an external support until full maturity has been attained.

Because the spine develops embryologically at the same time as the heart and genitourinary tract, a congenital scoliosis patient may have serious congenital anomalies throughout his body. Heart defects and congenital scoliosis have a 10 percent coincidence, whereas genitourinary abnormalities are seen in 17 percent of congenital scoliosis patients. Therefore, all congenital patients undergoing surgery should have an intravenous pyelogram and a myelogram along with a good cardiac examination.

NEUROFIBROMATOSIS AND OTHER TYPES OF SCOLIOSIS

Neurofibromatosis, described in Chapter 5, can lead to extremely severe spinal deformities consisting of scoliotic and kyphotic components (Fig. 5-11). These patients must also be protected by external means after spinal arthrodesis because in many instances the deforming condition remains until full maturation has been attained.

Mesenchymal scoliosis develops due to a specific connective tissue disorder such as Marfan's syndrome (Fig. 8-18), homocystinuria, and Ehlers-Danlos syndrome. These conditions can cause severely progressive curves and should be treated aggressively if the patient's general health permits.

Traumatic scoliosis can result from fractures or dislocations, laminectomy (as was mentioned in the section on spinal trauma), and irradiation. Often patients with Wilm's tumor or neuroblastoma undergo surgery or irradiation therapy through the involved lumbar region. Unfortunately, however, the x-ray

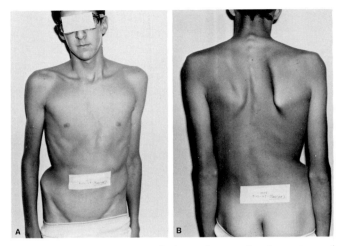

Fig. 8-18.   14-year-old boy with Marfan's syndrome, showing extreme height and double major curve. He also had arachnodactyly and high-arched palate. Although he wore glasses, he did not have dislocated lenses in his eyes. He responded well to brace treatment.

beam that destroys the tumor also has a devastating effect on the vertebral end plates and growth centers of the vertebrae on the side of the tumor. Patients receiving radiation therapy for such tumors many times develop marked scoliosis because growth centers on the irradiated side are destroyed (Fig. 8-19). The development of newer techniques, better therapeutic x-ray machines, and an awareness of epiphyseal damage has reduced this problem in the last few years.

The other types of scoliosis, such as osteochondro-dystrophies (Fig. 8-20), rheumatoid disease and metabolic conditions, will not be described individually in this text since they are less common causes of scoliosis, and our attention will be focused mainly on idiopathic, paralytic, and congenital types.

Spondyloytic scoliosis is due to nerve root irritation secondary to spondylolisthesis—most commonly at L-5 and the sacrum. As the vertebral slippage progresses forward on the sacrum, the first sacral nerve roots become stretched and cause a painful "list" and scoliosis to develop (Fig 8-21). The curve caused by spondylolytic scoliosis is usually C-shaped and spans the thoracic and entire lumbar spine directly to the sacrum.

The curve can usually be reduced by having the patient sit in a chair and bend his knees, thus relaxing the sciatic nerve. The curve also tends to resolve in the supine position. The best treatment is a spinal exploration, at which time the nerve roots are inspected and freed with a bilateral foraminotomy. A spinal fusion is then performed from L-4 to the sacrum, usually with complete relief of symptom and spontaneous correction of the scoliosis.

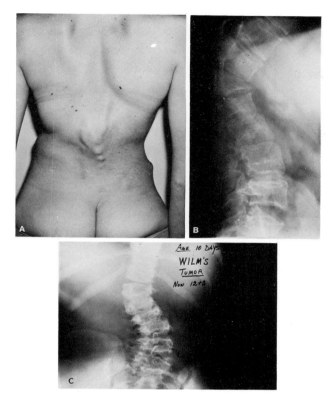

Fig. 8-19A.   12-year-old girl with Wilms' tumor first diagnosed at
10 days of age. X-ray treatment of tumor saved her life, but
irreversibly damaged vertebral end plates in lumbar spine. *B*.
Marked kyphosis, *C*. Lumbar scoliosis secondary to irradiation.

If the scoliosis is long standing, the curve may be structural and post-operative Milwaukee bracing may be required for some time. A herniated disc in an adolescent can cause a similar problem, with painful scoliosis and a list. Surgery is indicated if nonoperative measures fail (Fig. 8-22).

Thoracogenic scoliosis occurs after thoracoplasty or thoracotomy in the growing child, especially when a rib is removed. The concavity is usually on the side of the incision. In recent years more sternal splitting incisions have been used for heart surgery in children, and fewer cases of thoracogenic scoliosis are now occurring (Fig. 8-23).

Hysterical scoliosis can be extremely difficult to diagnose. It is particularly common in adolescent girls, usually because of psychological or psychiatric problems that lead them to develop unusual postural conditions. These generally are corrected under hypnosis or phenobarbital anesthesia. These

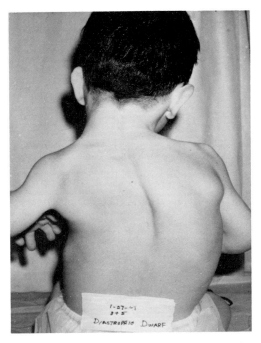

Fig. 8-20.   Severe right thoracolumbar scoliosis in a diastrophic dwarf whose family refused all treatment. He became paraplegic and died secondary to scoliosis.

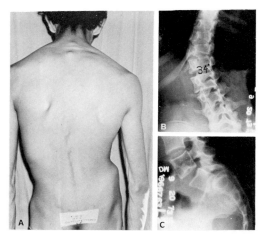

Fig. 8-21.   Spondylolytic scoliosis due to grade II spondylolisthesis of L-5. *A*. Marked list of patient; this disappeared in supine position. *B*. 34° left thoracolumbar scoliosis. *C*. Grade II spondylolisthesis of L-5 on sacrum.

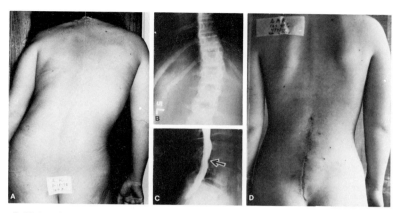

Fig. 8-22*A.* Scoliosis secondary to herniated disc; patient lists to right because of severe pain and muscle spasm. *B.* X-ray shows discogenic scoliosis. *C.* Myelogram outlines herniated disc at L-4 and 5. *D.* Patient 8 days postoperatively, after having sutures removed. Appearance is dramatically improved. All sciatic pain and muscle spasm had resolved, and patient's posture was practically normal. Disc excision at L-4 and 5 was performed, along with spine fusion from L-4 to sacrum.

patients differ from malingerers in that the hysterical component is subconscious, and the patient is not aware of any psychological cause of the problem. Psychiatric therapy often completely resolves the hysterical scoliosis (Fig. 8-24).

Functional scoliosis is secondary to postural deformities or a pelvic obliquity due to a short leg on one side. Some patients especially adolescents, have extremely poor posture (Fig. 8-25). Children seem to slouch and carry themselves in most peculiar attitudes and continue these same attitudes into their study habits at home or at school. Sometimes proper training by a good therapist in sitting, standing, and walking is needed before such a scoliosis can be resolved.

When scoliosis is due to an actual leg length discrepancy, scanograms can usually help to establish the problem, and an appropriate lift on one shoe can be of help. However, some patients have a pelvic obliquity due to a lumbar scoliosis, causing what seems to be a short leg (an "apparent" leg length discrepancy). In actuality, both legs are of equal length, but most patients with lumbar scoliosis do have a high-riding pelvis on the side of the concavity. All too frequently, an examining physician is unaware of the scoliosis and adds a shoe lift to the apparently short side, therefore increasing the pelvic obliquity and aggravating lumbar scoliosis. Patients with leg length discrepancies should be carefully evaluated to determine whether the discrepancy is actual or apparent, and then appropriate treatment should be instituted (Fig. 9-1B).

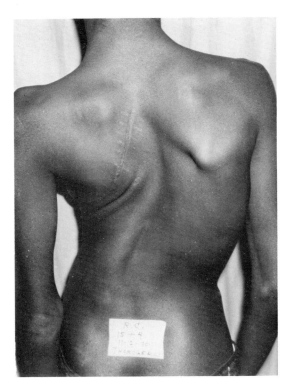

Fig. 8-23.   Thoracogenic scoliosis. Right thoracic scoliosis in a 15-year, 4-month-old boy who had thoractomy at 2 years of age for congenital heart disease. Scar is directly under scapula on left side. This type of scoliosis can be progressive, but incidence has been decreasing since sternal splitting incisions have been used more frequently in cardiac and thoracic surgery.

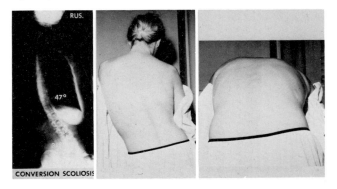

Fig. 8-24.   Hysterical scoliosis due to conversion reaction. Patient had left thoracolumbar scoliosis due to severe psychiatric problems. After psychiatric care, scoliosis resolved completely. (Courtesy Louis A. Goldstein, M.D.)

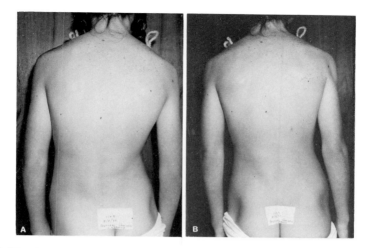

Fig. 8-25. Postural scoliosis and kyphosis in an 11-year, 9-month-old girl. Patient had obvious scoliotic deformity that concerned her parents. But, she could easily correct curvature upon command, and resolved completely both kyphosis and scoliosis after physiotherapy and muscle strengthening exercises. Exercises are useless in all other forms of scoliosis except when combined with Milwaukee bracing.

REFERENCES

1. Beals RK: Homocystinuria. A report of two cases and review of the literature. J Bone Joint Surg 51A:1564, 1969
2. Beals RK: Nosologic and genetic aspects of scoliosis. Clin Orthop 93:23–32, 1973
3. Beighton PH, Horan F: Orthopaedic aspects of the Ehlers-Danlos syndrome. J Bone Joint Surg 51B:444, 1969
4. Bjorksten J: The cross-linkage theory of aging. J Am Geriatr Soc 16:408, 1968
5. Bjure J, Nachemson A: Non-treated scoliosis, Clin Orthop 93:44–52, 1973
6. Brenton DP, Dow CJ, James JIP, et al: Homocystinuria and Marfan's syndrome. A comparison. J Bone Joint Surg 54B:277–297, 1972
7. Brooks L, Gerberg E, Mazur H, et al.: The epidemiology of Scoliosis—a prospective study. J Bone Joint Surg 55A:436, 1973
8. Collis D, Ponseti I: Long-term follow-up of patients with idiopathic scoliosis not treated surgically. J Bone Joint Surg 51A:425, 1969
9. Cowell HR, Hall JN, MacEwen GD: Genetic aspects of idiopathic scoliosis. Clin Orthop 86:121, 1972
10. DeGeorge F, Fischer R: Idiopathic scoliosis: genetic and environmental aspects. J Med Genet 4:251, 1967
11. Enneking WF, Harrington P: Pathological changes in scoliosis. J Bone Joint Surg 51A:165, 1969
12. Garret AL, Perry J, Nickel UL: Paralytic scoliosis. Clin Orthop 21:117, 1961
13. Goldstein LA, Waugh TR: Classification and terminology in scoliosis. Clin Orthop 93:10–22, 1973

14. Hibbs R: A report of fifty-nine cases of scoliosis treated by the fusion operation. J Bone Joint Surg 22:3, 1924

15. James J: Scoliosis Edinburgh & London, Livingstone, 1967

16. Kane W, Moe J: A scoliosis-prevalence survey in Minnesota. Clin Orthop 69:216, 1970

17. Katzman H, Waugh T, Berdon W: Skeletal changes following irradiation of childhood tumors. J Bone Joint Surg 51A:825, 1969

18. MacEwen GD: Personal communication

19. MacEwen GD, Cowell HR: Familial incidence of idiopathic scoliosis and its implications in patient treatment. J Bone Joint Surg 52A:405, 1970

20. Nachemson A: A long-term follow-up study of non-treated scoliosis. Acta Orthop Scand 39:466, 1968

21. Nilsonne V, Lundgren KD: Long-term prognosis in idiopathic scoliosis. Acta Orthop Scand 39:456, 1968

22. Ponseti IV: The pathogenesis of adolescent scoliosis, in Zorab P (ed): Proceedings of a Second Symposium on Scoliosis. Edinburgh & London, Livingstone, 1968

23. Ponseti IV: Skeletal lesions produced by aminonitriles. Clin Orthop 9:131, 1957

24. Roth A, Rosenthal A, Hall JE, et al: Scoliosis and congenital heart disease. Clin Orthop 93:95–102, 1973

25. Shands A Jr, Eisberg H: The incidence of scoliosis in the state of Delaware: A Study of 50,000 minifilms of the chest made during a survey for tuberculosis. J Bone Joint Surg 37A:1243, 1955

26. Sinex FM: Cross-linkage and aging. Adv Gerontol Res 1:165, 1964

27. Urbaniak JR, Stelling FH: Progression of the scoliotic curve after completion of the excursion of the iliac epiphysis. A preliminary report. J Bone Joint Surg 51A:205, 1969

28. Winter RB: Congenital scoliosis. Clin Orthop 93:75–94, 1973

29. Wynne-Davies R: Familial (idiopathic) scoliosis. A family survey. J Bone Joint Surg 50B:24, 1968

30. Zorab PA: Total hydroxyproline excretion in scoliosis, in Zorab P (ed): Proceedings of a Second Symposium on Scoliosis. Edinburgh & London, Livingstone, 1968

9
Clinical and Roentgenographic Evaluation of the Scoliosis Patient

Although scoliosis may play a relatively small role in the average orthopedist's practice, it is a difficult condition to treat. One reason is that scoliosis is an emotionally charged condition. Parents usually have severe guilt feelings because they feel that they have neglected their child. They feel even worse when they learn that most cases of idiopathic scoliosis have a genetic basis, and that they "gave" it to their child. In addition, parents learn that the earlier scoliosis is diagnosed, the better it can be treated. This usually leads to hostility—justified or not—against the family physician or pediatrician for not noticing the curvature in his routine office or camp physical.

Often by the time the family reaches the orthopedist's office they are confused, angry, and frightened. It is important for the orthopedist to remember that he is first of all a physician. He must use great tact in his initial interview, since those golden moments may make the difference between proper acceptance or total rejection of treatment by the patient and family.

The patient is usually a teen-age girl in a difficult stage of her life. In addition to the many hormonal changes she is going through, she must now cope mentally and socially with what she and her family consider a disaster.

During the initial examination it is important not to criticize prior treatment or the delay of it, since this only adds to the sense of guilt and defeat already present. If the humanistic and optimistic approach is used, long-lasting bonds will be made with the family and establish the groundwork for the years of treatment and follow-up that lie ahead. Since orthopedic care of the scoliosis patient frequently extends over a prolonged time and may involve spinal bracing, casting, or surgery, thorough office examination is important. Recommendations based on x-ray findings alone or after casual examination should be discouraged. The orthopedic surgeon must understand the fundamentals of scoliosis to perform a meaningful examination. A plan of examination is advantageous and should consist of the patient being gowned by a nurse who records vital signs, such as standing and sitting heights and weight. A history is then obtained with the parents and child present. During this time, continuous observation of the child's reactions and feelings is an aid in prescribing appropriate subsequent treatment.

Obtaining a detailed history from the parents with the patient present can bring out many interesting subtleties. Most adolescents reveal that the scoliosis was first noted by a friend, gym teacher, dressmaker, or one of their parents while on vacation. These patients rarely complain of pain, but questioning about backache or tiredness may uncover symptoms that they had related to some other incident.

Any reported pain should be evaluated since it may lead to a diagnosis of spinal cord tumor or bony anomaly such as osteoid osteoma. The physician should inquire whether lung x-rays were taken during the previous 6 or 12 months, since curve progression is easier to evaluate if these records are available. A thorough past medical history frequently uncovers such conditions as eye problems or hernias that could be related to Marfan's syndrome. Most children do not have a cardiorespiratory history, but if they do, this indicates that the scoliosis is rapidly progressing or is of neuromuscular origin.

The physical examination is then performed with both parents present. Many adolescent girls are so modest that their parents have not seen or examined their backs for months or even years. Most fathers have not seen the deformity before, and they should be encouraged to remain in the examining room—the patient is specifically requested to allow the father to do so.

A good general physical examination is mandatory. The appearance of secondary sexual characteristics and height comparisons with siblings and parents can indicate future growth patterns. The skin should be carefully examined for café-au-lait markings and the general neuromuscular development of the patient noted. The entire spine should be examined for areas of pigment or hair patches, which can lead to the identification of spinal dysraphism. Cardiopulmonary status can be examined easily using a portable office spirometer, although this device is not as accurate as sophisticated hospital breathing equipment. Chest expansion, genitourinary status, and gait should be recorded, since these are often affected in congenital conditions. If the patient wears glasses, the eyes should be examined for dislocated lenses, which are common in Marfan's syndrome.

After the general examination, the entire trunk is examined. Trunk alignment is determined by dropping a plumb line from the base of the occiput to see whether the spine is level and in plumb or out of balance. Normally, the head is exactly over the gluteal cleft, and this is so in many double major curves (Fig. 9-1A). However, single major curves—especially thoracolumbar curves—usually throw the spine markedly out of alignment.

The patient is then told to bend forward and touch the ground, keeping his knees perfectly straight. The arms should hang straight in an attempt to touch the floor. Scapular prominence can be detected by placing a straight edge or spirit level directly above the rib prominence and measuring any difference between rib height on the concave side (Fig. 9-2A). Asymmetry of the neck line for cervical and high thoracic curves is best detected with the patient standing at ease.

Arm span from the tips of the middle fingers is used to measure accurately the vital capacity. Since scoliosis patients are much shorter than normal because of their condition, vital capacity should not be based on their standing height, which will distort normal base values. A proper formula has been evolved to measure what should be normal respiratory volume based on arm span from the tips of the index fingers.

The patient's curve should then be assessed and right and left erect side-bending attempted. This indicates spinal flexibility and the potential degree of correction (Fig. 8-3). Applying direct pressure over the apex of the curve is also helpful in obtaining this information, and having an aide lift the patient gently by the head also reflects elasticity and correction potential in the vertebral column.

Shoulder inequality should be carefully measured, along with anterior rib or breast asymmetry. Many mothers are very concerned that one breast, usually on the convex side, is smaller than the other. They incorrectly feel that one breast has not grown at the same rate as the other. But this discrepancy is due to distortion of the ribs underlying the breast tissue and not to an actual diminution or lack of development of one breast.

The physician must carefully assess pelvic obliquity, which can be non-structural because of a short leg or habit pattern, or structural, due to contracture of the muscle groups above or below the pelvic crests. In neuromuscular scoliosis, there is almost always an associated pelvic obliquity that may be fixed or correctable and can be properly assessed during the initial examination. Actual leg length should be measured from the anterior superior iliac spine to the medial malleolus at the ankle and compared to apparent leg length measured from the umbilicus to the ankle. Since leg lengths can vary greatly, this measurement is important to differentiate actual leg length discrepancy from an apparent one due to pelvic obliquity (Fig. 9-1B).

After determining leg length, the physician should make a brief but thorough neuromuscular examination. All reflexes, sensation, and motor power are carefully recorded. In children with congenital conditions, sensory or motor loss is often the first indication of a congenital spinal defect. As

Fig. 9-1. Clinical evaluation of scoliosis patient. *A.* Measurement of spine to check balance. Plumb line dropped from vertebra prominens (7 cervical vertebra) deviates toward side that is out of balance. *B.* Measurement of actual and apparent leg length. Scoliosis patients usually have pelvic obliquity, especially true in lumbar scoliosis where pelvic crest is higher on concave side. This causes an apparent leg length discrepancy, but actually legs are of equal length. By measuring actual leg length from anterior superior iliac spine to medial malleolus on both sides, we can tell if leg length difference is due to actual shortening of one leg. Apparent leg length discrepancy due to pelvic obliquity is corrected by proper spinal bracing. Sometimes a shoe lift can be added on the apparently longer leg, never the shorter one. In severe cases, pelvic obliquity must be corrected surgically.

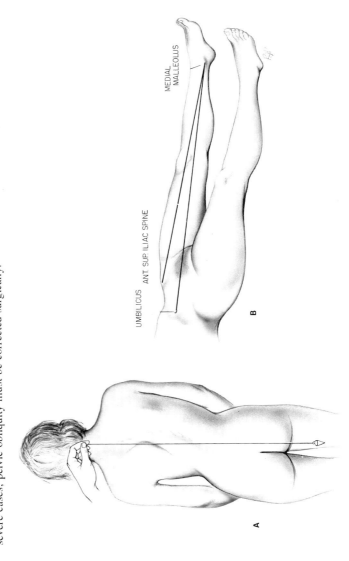

UMBILICUS ANT SUP ILIAC SPINE

MEDIAL
MALLEOLUS

A

B

128

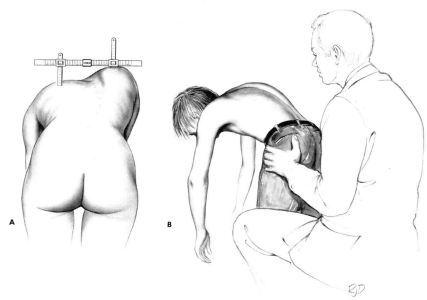

Fig. 9-2.   Clinical evaluation of rib deformity and vertebral rotation. *A*. As patient bends forward, examiner places straight edge with spirit level in center across patient's rib hump to determine difference between both sides of thoracic cage. Lower side is then measured (in cm) and defined as rib valley. *B*. Siblings can be screened easily by having patient undress to waist and bend forward so that entire spinal area can be viewed.

mentioned in the section on spinal dysraphism, it is important to examine the feet and watch the patient's gait, since a varus heel or cavus foot may be due to a spinal cord tumor or diastematomyelia. In all cases of neuromuscular or congenital scoliosis, the stability of the hips should be carefully evaluated. Many of these patients have congenital dislocations or subluxations that may not have been previously identified, but which could be serious if treatment includes any type of traction procedure, especially skeletal traction. In patients with obvious myelomeningocele, all functioning muscles and sensory dermatomes must be carefully examined and accurately recorded, preferably by more than one examiner.

   If at all possible, the examination should include clinical photographs, especially with views to assess the patient's rib hump on forward bending. These photographs can be taken with a Polaroid camera and can be invaluable in providing follow-up care and in assessing the results of treatment.

   The patient's siblings must be examined also since so much idiopathic scoliosis is familial and many early cases can be identified in this manner (Fig. 9-2B). Also, parents should be advised that other relatives, such as nephews and nieces, could have scoliosis, and that they should contact other family members to be certain that all adolescent relatives are screened adequately. It is not wise to emphasize scoliosis existing in the parents since late recognition of this condition only enhances parents' guilt complex and does not aid in treatment.

After thorough examination, the physician studies available x-rays, and measures the curves. These are correlated with the patient's physical deformity, and the family is then explained the cause of scoliosis and the appropriate means of treatment.

RADIOGRAPHIC ASSESSMENT OF THE SCOLIOSIS PATIENT

Most patients arrive for examination with a stack of x-rays, many of which are of little value in properly assessing the patient. Since parents today are so concerned with x-ray exposure, it is judicious to take only those films that will give specific meaning to the scoliosis examination. For each new scoliosis patient, it is best to obtain anteroposterior views of the thoracic and lumbar spine in the standing and supine positions. A lateral view of the thoracic and lumbar spine is then taken in the standing position, along with a spot lateral of L-5 and S-1 also in the erect position.

It is desirable to obtain the films on a 14 × 36 inch cassette because this will permanently record all vertebrae from the occiput to the sacrum, even on large children and adults. However, most x-ray departments are not equipped to process or handle these long cassettes, and then 14 × 17 inch films must be used. With a 14 × 17 inch film, it is essential that the iliac crest on both sides be well visualized, along with the base of the occiput. Side-bending films are taken only preoperatively in the hospital to determine which segment of the spine to fuse; nonstructural curves do not need fusion.

Some physicians prefer to take an A-P x-ray of the left hand and wrist to compare with the Gruelich and Pyle atlas to determine bone age. However, bone age can usually be assessed even more accurately by evaluating the spine films of the iliac crests and vertebral rings, especially in the thoracolumbar junction. If the Gruelich and Pyle atlas is used, the actual bone age can be determined in contrast to the patient's chronologic age; these ages often differ in adolescents. In certain ethnic and racial groups, maturation is complete by age 13 or 14, whereas in other racial groups the age of maturation is 18 to 20.

Always be certain to include in the initial examination the spot films of L-5 and S-1 in the erect position, since spondylolisthesis and spondylolysis occur in 5 percent of the general population and are also present in the same percentage in the scoliosis population. The presence of spondylolisthesis may greatly alter the treatment plan for a specific patient, and this condition must be diagnosed at the onset of treatment.

X-rays for scoliosis have classically been measured by one of two methods. The initial Risser-Ferguson method has been essentially discarded because it lacks accuracy and reproducibility among groups of examiners. It is described briefly for the sake of completeness, but should be used only in certain types of congenital scoliosis for which the favored Cobb method cannot be used.

Both methods of measurement are based on determinations of upper and lower end vertebrae. The end vertebrae, at the upper and lower ends of the curve, are those which have maximum tilting toward the concavity of the curve. In other words, the superior end vertebra is the last vertebra in which the superior border points toward the concavity of the curve to be measured. The inferior end vertebra is the last one whose inferior border points toward the concavity of the curve being measured.

In the Risser-Ferguson method, small dots are placed in the centers of the upper and lower end vertebrae. In addition, a small dot is placed in the center of the apical vertebra, which is the vertebra with the most wedging and deformity and is at the apex of the curve. Straight lines are then drawn from the dot in each end vertebra through the dot in the apical vertebra, and the intersecting angle is measured with a protractor (Fig. 9-3).

The Cobb method is easily mastered by repeated practice and consists of drawing a horizontal line along the superior border of the superior end vertebra. Another horizontal line is then drawn along the inferior border of the inferior end vertebra with perpendicular lines being erected from each of the horizontal lines. The intersecting angle produced is then measured. The Cobb method gives larger angles than the Risser-Ferguson technique, and correction can more easily be compared with the former method during treatment and follow-up (Fig. 9-3). The Cobb technique is advocated by the Scoliosis Research Society, which classifies all forms of scoliosis in one of seven groups—group 1: curves 0–20°; group 2: curves 21–30°; group 3: curves 31–50°; group 4: curves 51–75°; group 5: curves 76–100°; group 6: curves 101–125°; group 7: curves 126° and above.

Vertebral rotation is inherent in scoliosis. It forces the ribs on the convex side backward, thus elevating the scapula in the thoracic curve, with its resultant cosmetic deformity. There are two methods of measuring rotation; one is based on the deviation of the spinous process from the midline. Since spinous processes can be easily misshapen in various types of curves, this method is not generally used. The second, more accurate, method of evaluating rotation consists of examining pedicles of the most rotated vertebral body. If the vertebra with its pedicles rotates so that one pedicle is in the center of the body of the vertebra, this is called 3+ rotation (Fig. 9-4).

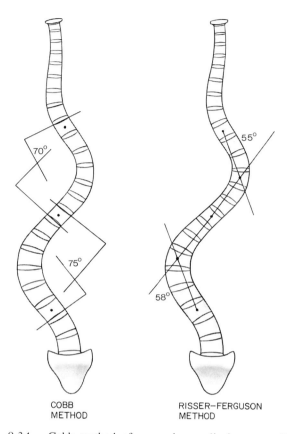

COBB
METHOD

RISSER–FERGUSON
METHOD

Fig. 9-3A. Cobb method of measuring scoliosis x-rays. End vertebrae are located first. Upper end vertebra is last vertebra whose superior border points toward concavity of curve. Lowest end vertebra of upper curve to be measured is last vertebra whose inferior border points toward concavity of curve. Perpendicular lines are then erected from lines which have been drawn parallel to the end vertebrae and the intersecting angle measured. The vertebra between two curves is called the "apical vertebra". B. The Risser–Ferguson method is based on placing a small dot in the center of the end vertebrae and in the center of the apical vertebra. The intersecting angle is then measured. This technique is reserved primarily for certain types of congenital curves where the Cobb technique cannot be efficiently used.

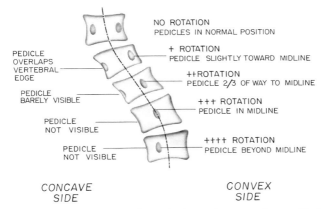

NO ROTATION
PEDICLES IN NORMAL POSITION

PEDICLE
OVERLAPS
VERTEBRAL
EDGE

+ ROTATION
PEDICLE SLIGHTLY TOWARD MIDLINE

++ROTATION
PEDICLE 2/3 OF WAY TO MIDLINE

PEDICLE
BARELY VISIBLE

+++ ROTATION
PEDICLE IN MIDLINE

PEDICLE
NOT VISIBLE

PEDICLE
NOT VISIBLE

++++ ROTATION
PEDICLE BEYOND MIDLINE

*CONCAVE
SIDE*

*CONVEX
SIDE*

Fig. 9-4. Measurement of vertebral rotation according to Nash andMoe is based on deviation of pedicles of vertebral bodies as they rotate. A vertebral body in which convex-sided pedicle has rotated toward midline is identified as 3+ rotation.

Consistent use of exactly the same radiographic examining techniques can give much more meaningful information to subsequent examiners, since they are then all speaking the same language. Determination of maturation in adolescent patients is extremely important, even thouugh scoliosis can progress throughout a patient's adult life. Generally, in girls growth ceases and maturation is complete by age 18, whereas boys usually mature 12 to 18 months later. Knowing the approximate time of full maturation is important because in most cases scoliosis progression slows (but does not stop) significantly when the patient is fully mature.

Maturation is difficult to judge, and many accumulated facts aid in determining it. Observation of the child's parents and siblings can help in estimating how tall the child will probably grow. Also, as mentioned before, certain racial and ethnic groups are known for short or tall stature. In girls, the date of menarche and the acquisition of secondary sexual characteristics, such as breast development and pubic and axillary hair growth, are also helpful in assessing maturation. Finally, a review of the patient's x-rays can be coupled with the Gruelich and Pyle evaluation of the left hand and wrist.

The erect and supine A-P x-rays of the thoracic and lumbar spine provide important information. A patient whose erect film measures 45° by the Cobb method but whose curve reduces to 30° on supine positioning still has an extremely flexible spine, which is bound to continue to curve regardless of the patient's chronological age. Risser originally described excursion of the iliac crests as a means of determining skeletal maturation. Although this technique is helpful, it must be coupled with all of the other facts of maturation to make a reasonably educated guess as to the patient's skeletal age. When the iliac epiphysis is completely across from the lateral to the medial side near the sacroiliac joint, and the epiphyseal plate has disappeared along with early fusion of the epiphysis to the pelvic wall, maturation can be said to be complete. Maturation can be assessed more accuratley by observing the vertebral ring apophyses or end plates. These are best seen in the thoracic and lumbar regions, and maturation usually is complete when the ring apophysis has completely united to the vertebral body (Fig. 9-5).

In 1972, Mehta studied the radiographic assessment of the rib-vertebral angle in infantile scoliosis. The angle formed by the junction of the ribs with the spine was measured in the thoracic region of 138 children with infantile idiopathic scoliosis under the age of 2. By assessing the rib-vertebral angle at the apex of the curve and observing the relationship of the head of the rib to the body of the vertebra in anteroposterior radiographs, Mehta was able to predict accurately which curves would progress and which were likely to resolve. This technique is an aid to prognosis in infantile idiopathic scoliosis but does not seem to apply to juvenile or adolescent scoliosis. So far, we have found no good method of predicting curve progression or resolution in these age groups. A radiographic technique or laboratory test to determine which curves are likely to progress would be of great prognostic significance and would allay a great deal of parental anxiety.

PULMONARY PHYSIOLOGY IN THE SCOLIOSIS PATIENT

Cardiopulmonary problems are rare in patients with curves less than 60° Cobb. Nevertheless, pulmonary changes must be assessed accurately as scoliosis increases, especially when surgery is contemplated. As the Cobb measurement increases, rotation also progresses with narrowing of the chest cavity on the convex side with decreasing room for lung expansion. Thoracic and thoracolumbar curves are likely to cause advancing respiratory restriction in later life. In severe scoliotic deformities, premature death is usually due to respiratory disease, superimposed pneumonia, and/or cor pulmonale.

Total lung capacity (TLC) is generally considered the sum of the residual volume (RV) or the air left in the lungs after a forced expiration, and the vital capacity (VC), or the amount of air available for respiratory exchange. In scoliosis the pulmonary deficit is due to "restrictive disease" because of distortion of the rib cage as well as cardiomegaly. There is little change in the RV, but the VC is severely reduced in direct proportion to the magnitude of the scoliotic curve. Therefore, the TLC is decreased, and as the patient becomes older he develops chronic emphysema, especially if he smokes. Smoking can cause an increase in residual volume, which continues to reduce total lung capacity (Fig. 9-6).

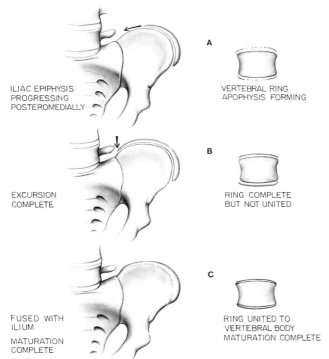

ILIAC EPIPHYSIS
PROGRESSING
POSTEROMEDIALLY

A

VERTEBRAL RING
APOPHYSIS FORMING

EXCURSION
COMPLETE

B

RING COMPLETE
BUT NOT UNITED

FUSED WITH
ILIUM

MATURATION
COMPLETE

C

RING UNITED TO
VERTEBRAL BODY
MATURATION COMPLETE

Fig. 9-5.   Radiographic assessment of spinal maturation. Iliac crest generally starts to form anterolaterally and progresses toward sacroiliac joint. When crest begins to mature, several years of spinal maturation remain, no matter how tall child may be. Spinal growth cannot be complete until iliac crest is completely fused with ilium, and even then scoliosis curves can progress throughout adult life. A more accurate method of determining when scoliosis curve will stop progressing rapidly is to measure vertebral ring apophyses. When apophyses, especially in thoracic spine, are noted to have united with vertebral body, maturation is complete.

Additionally, the blood distributed to the areas of the lungs that are being ventilated and the air distributed to those same areas being perfused causes a relationship known as the ventilation-perfusion ratio, or the V/Q ratio. ''V'' is the ventilation per minute and ''Q'' is the perfusion per minute in that portion of the lung under consideration. In the erect patient, the ventilation-perfusion ratio is heavily weighted in favor of ventilation in the upper lung area, and perfusion occurs mainly in the lower area.

In a scoliosis patient with atelectasis or pneumonia, perfusion occurs in the

NORMAL FOR THIS PATIENT	SEVERE SCOLIOSIS
BLOOD GASES	
O_2 TENSION ....80– 90 mm. Hg	.... 68.4 mm. Hg
CO_2 TENSION............................ 37–40 mm. Hg	.... 50.8 mm. Hg
O_2 SATURATION........................ 95+ %	.... 91.5 %
pH 7.40	.... 7.39
LUNG VOLUME	
VITAL CAPACITY........................ 2.98 L	.... 0.90 L
RESIDUAL VOLUME .... 1.05 L	.... 0.50 L
TOTAL LUNG CAPACITY............. 4.03 L } ± 20 %	.... 1.40 L
FUNCTIONAL RESIDUAL CAPACITY .... 1.68 L	.... 0.30 L
MECHANICS OF BREATHING	
FORCED EXPIRATORY VOLUME FIRST SECOND .... 2.47 L ± 20 %	..............0.65 L
BLOOD-GAS DISTRIBUTION	
ALVEOLAR ARTERY pO_2 DIFFERENTIAL .... 10mm.Hg ± 50 %	.... 29 mm. Hg
PHSIOLOGIC DEAD SPACE........ 35 % ± 20 %	.... 30 %

AGE: 16 YEARS   WEIGHT: 35 KILOGRAMS
HEIGHT: 1.38 METERS (BASED ON ARM SPAN)

Fig. 9-6.   Pulmonary function chart for 16-year-old girl weighing 35 kg with a height of 1.38 m (based on arm span). Norm for this type of patient is on left side of figure. Patient of same age, height, and weight who has severe scoliosis will develop marked pulmonary restriction and compromise as indicated on right.

unventilated portions of the lungs, leading to a shunt of blood from the right to the left side of the heart. The V/Q ratio falls, causing anoxia. In the patient with severe scoliosis and advancing age, alveolar ventilation is decreased and arterial levels of high pCO_2, low pH, and low pO_2 occur. This usually causes death due to cor pulmonale, pneumonia, or both (Fig. 9-7).

There have been many reports in the literature that corrective surgery for severely scoliotic patients does not really increase the vital capacity. This may be true, but recent studies using radioactive xenon have shown that ventilation-perfusion ratios actually are increased and that more sophisticated measuring devices are needed to show that pulmonary function is improved after operative correction. Patients who have undergone surgery readily tell their physicians that they can now accomplish much more than they previously could. Also, patients in pulmonary failure who have undergone surgery have been able to live additional years with little pulmonary difficulty.

The most obvious, but by no means the only, pulmonary abnormality in

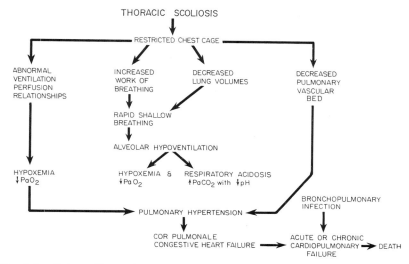

Fig. 9-7. Schema illustrating sequence of events after progressive increase in thoracic scoliosis, generally in curves over 60°. The more severe the curve, generally, the greater will be the patient's respiratory difficulty. (Courtesy James P. Smith, M.D)

scoliosis is the reduction of lung volume. There is relatively little reduction of residual volume and a disproportionately severe decrease in expiratory reserve volume, which is typical of paralytic patients. The expected values of normal pulmonary function can be derived by arm span measured from the index fingertips according to a formula by Westgate (armspan divided by 1.03 equals corrected height).

The most direct line of evidence presently available which indicates improvement in pulmonary function after surgery has been described by Shannon and Reisborough. These investigators demonstrated a significant increase in arterial oxygen tension in patients with idiopathic curves greater than 60° Cobb. This was associated with a decrease in the volume of "wasted ventilation" (that portion of the tidal volume which does not participate in gas exchange; includes gas in anatomic dead space as well as that distributed to nonperfused or poorly perfused alveolar units). Considered in light of concomitant increase in arterial oxygen tension and no significant change in vital capacity, tidal volume, or respiratory frequency, the only adequate explanation for the observed decrease in the volume of wasted ventilation is redistribution of ventilation, or, more likely, redistribution of both ventilation and perfusion after surgery so as to effect overall a more favorable ventilation-perfusion relationship.

REFERENCES

1. Calvo IJ: Observations on the growth of the female adolescent spine and its relation to scoliosis. Clin Orthop 10:40, 1957
2. Cobb JR: The problem of the primary curve. J Bone Joint Surg 42A:1413, 1960
3. Duval-Beaupére G: Pathogenic relationships between scoliosis and growth, in Zorab P (ed): Scoliosis and Growth, Proceedings of a Third Symposium on Scoliosis. Edinburgh and London, Livingstone, 1971, p. 58
4. Greulich WW, Pyle SI: Radiographic Atlas of Skeletal Development of the Hand and Wrist, ed 2. California, Stanford University Press, 1959
5. Hoppenfeld S: Pre-operative evaluation of the scoliotic patient, in Keim H (ed): Second Annual Post-Graduate Course on the Management and Care of the Scoliosis Patient. Warsaw, Indiana, Zimmer, 1970, p 5
6. Levine DB: Orthopaedic evaluation of the scoliosis patient, in Keim H (ed): Third Annual Post-Graduate Course on the Management and Care of the Scoliosis Patient. Warsaw, Indiana, Zimmer, 1971, p. 7
7. Metha MH: The rib-vertebral angle in the early diagnosis between resolving and progressive infantile scoliosis. J Bone Joint Surg 54B:230–243, 1972
8. Nash CL Jr, Moe JH: A study of vertebral rotation. J Bone Joint Surg 51A:223, 1969
9. Smith JP: Pulmonary evaluation of the scoliosis patient, in Keim H (ed): Third Annual Post-Graduate Course on the Management and Care of the Scoliosis Patient. Warsaw, Indiana, Zimmer, 1971, p 32
10. Westgate HD: Pulmonary function in thoracic scoliosis before and after corrective surgery. Minn Med 53:839, 1970

10

Nonoperative Treatment for Scoliosis

Treatment of scoliosis dates back at least to the Stone Age. Carvings on cave walls, as well as woodcuts from thousands of years ago, indicate that man has been aware of the devastating anatomical and cosmetic deformities of scoliosis for centuries. Over the years, hundreds of attempts were made to correct the spine, usually with little permanent effect. The earliest forms of nonoperative treatment were those in which the patient was hung from a harness or placed in a prone position and stretched by both the head and feet. Sometimes "therapists" actually walked on the patient's hump in an effort to reduce it.

Spinal bracing was first attempted during the Middle Ages when the wealthy social groups, mostly kings and members of their courts, instructed armorers to mold metal corsets in an attempt to halt scoliosis progression. Unfortunately, these were merely passive devices and did not incorporate any active corrective principle. It was not until 1945 that Blount and Schmidt developed a brace that was the culmination of many years of attempts at brace control to correct scoliosis and kyphosis.

The present Milwaukee brace is a streamlined, modern version of the original device with which Blount and Schmidt started their crusade for nonoperative treatment. The road was difficult and many obstacles, such as physicians' skepticism and patients' rejection, had to be overcome. In most civilized countries, the Milwaukee brace is now considered an extremely important form of correction for scoliosis and a valuable adjunct in certain cases where bracing and surgery are combined to obtain the desired end result. A properly constructed and well-fitted Milwaukee brace undoubtedly will help the average scoliosis patient.

The patient and his family must cooperate and the patient must want to wear the brace if the spine is to be corrected. American children have learned to accept braces on their teeth, and braces have actually become a status symbol, especially in the more affluent suburbs of America. The Milwaukee brace probably will never achieve such social status, but it is certainly much more important cosmetically and functionally to have a straight painless back than to have even teeth. Many of my patients have worn orthodontic appliances for several years and their parents have spent thousands of dollars for a proper bite and pleasing cosmetic appearance. When the Milwaukee brace is suggested, there are usually initial signs of rejection in the entire family. Most families do not understand how important a properly balanced spine can be for the years that lie ahead. In speaking with parents, I usually employ the analogy that the spine must be in balance during adult life just as a car's tires must be in balance. If the front wheels of an auto are out of alignment, the entire chassis shakes and vibrates, so eventually the car rattles and does not last as long as an automobile in proper alignment.

Our spines are similar. The head should be directly over the pelvis, and the facet joints should be lined up so that there are no rotational deformities to invite osteoarthritic changes in adult life. All men who deal with scoliosis patients see the severe problems adults encounter when their spines have been out of balance for many years and severe vertebral rotation has been allowed to persist. These patients end up having low back pain of a mechanical nature that can cause disability and loss of work during a person's most productive age.

MILWAUKEE BRACE

Effectiveness

In my practice I estimate that the Milwaukee brace is effective in approximately 90 percent of all properly selected brace patients. If I place 100 properly chosen patients in Milwaukee braces, approximately 60 of them will have a significant reduction of the initial curvature, which can be held and maintained until full maturation. In another 30, the original scoliosis will be only slightly reduced, but their curves can be kept from progressing further during bracing. If these patients are held until full maturity and are then judiciously weaned from the brace, they many times hold a good final correction.

Approximately 10 percent of scoliosis patients have had such a severe genetic dose of scoliosis that they develop what we call malignant scoliosis. These patients are genetically destined to develop extremely severe curves that seem to continue no matter what form of nonoperative treatment is used. Many of these curves continue to progress even though the patient is properly treated with a Milwaukee brace, and when this is obvious to the physician in a child mature enough for spinal surgery (usually after a bone age of 12), surgery should be performed immediately.

These facts are explained to the family before prescribing a Milwaukee brace so that a good relationship can be maintained if the final result is not what the family anticipated. There is no way to predict whether a curve will respond successfully to bracing. Usually a tipoff that bracing will not work is a curve with severe rotational deformity in its major components and also a patient with a strong family history of scoliosis. Even in malignant curves, however, scoliosis can be adequately controlled in young patients until their spines have matured sufficiently to allow proper surgical correction. In this case, the brace has been valuable in keeping the patient's spine from developing the severe curves previously seen in juvenile and young adolescent patients before the advent of the Milwaukee brace.

Construction

The Milwaukee brace must be constructed by a well-trained orthotist. Not every orthotist can make a good Milwaukee brace. In fact, there are probably no more than 40 or 50 experts in constructing the Milwaukee brace in the United States. Many of the Milwaukee braces constructed should not bear the name Milwaukee brace—these are an insult to the ingenuity and principles Blount and Schmidt originally proposed (Figs. 10-1, 10-2).

A brace that is not made to the correct standards and is not properly prescribed by the physician will fail. The brace should not be blamed if it was not correctly used any more than a surgical technique should be blamed if it is poorly carried out by an unskilled surgeon. The greatest single error in Milwaukee bracing is to expect the brace to do the impossible. I often see patients who were braced for rapidly advancing 55° or 60° curves; such poor patient selection dooms the result to failure. One must always select the treatment to suit the individual patient and not try to force the patient into a treatment regimen.

In order to accomplish good spinal bracing, a team approach must be used. This team should consist of the orthopedic surgeon, the orthotist, a physiotherapist, and, in some instances, a social worker. This basic team should see all patients when they are examined since many physical and social problems can be treated adequately in group form, especially if all Milwaukee brace patients are seen in a clinic setting so that they can meet each other and find out that they are not the only ones in the world who have scoliosis and have to wear a brace. On Saturday mornings 50 to 60 patients congregate at our brace clinic to discuss various social and personal problems with each other and with other parents. These sessions are extremely effective in helping the patient

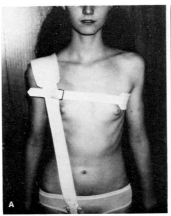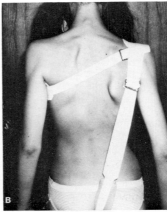

Fig. 10-1.   Patient treated for scoliosis with sling. One sling goes directly through groin, which caused considerable discomfort. In addition, she had right thoracic curve, and sling on right side was pulling down on the shoulder, not correcting scapular winging and causing rather marked left lumbar curve. Slings and makeshift arrangements never are of value in treating scoliosis and often delay appropriate treatment until only surgery can help the patient.

overcome shyness and discover that many other kids have similar and more serious problems. Psychologically, this experience is uplifting and rewarding to the patient and her family.

A properly prescribed, constructed, and fitted Milwaukee brace is unquestionably of great value in scoliosis management. An exercise program is also extremely effective and must be followed daily by the patient, both in and out of the brace. Exercises *alone* for scoliosis do little more than strengthen the patient's spine and never correct scoliosis!

I have seen many young patients who originally had curves ranging up to 30° and were told not to start any kind of exercise program but to return in 3 months. At least 20 percent of these patients have had permanent spontaneous remission of their scoliosis without any treatment whatsoever. If all of these patients had been placed on vigorous exercise programs, they would probably have signed sworn documents that the exercises made their scoliotic curves decrease or disappear. We do not understand why curves spontaneously resolve, but it does occur in a significant proportion of juvenile and adolescent scoliotics. The important factor to note is that a patient will get better or worse, depending on the inherited makeup, and exercises do nothing to change that genetic composition.

It has been well established, however, that exercises coupled with the Milwaukee brace are extremely effective. The patient's spine is immobilized in the brace and deossifies and softens with osteoporotic changes unless dynamic

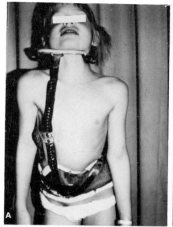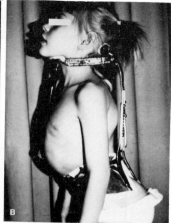

Fig. 10-2.   An improperly made brace which caused a jaw deformity by pressing upward on both sides of mandible. Brace does not fit patient—pelvic girdle is too small, and brace has caused lumbar lordosis. Poor brace-making causes lack of acceptance of brace techniques and results in certain failure.

exercises are undertaken to improve and maintain muscle tone and cause active curve correction. When this is done, the active effect of the Milwaukee brace continues to exert itself, and curves usually improve.

Advantages

The Milwaukee brace has many advantages over previous forms of brace therapy for scoliosis. It allows the patient ''active'' correction of the deformity; it allows freedom of motion and rarely interferes with social activity during treatment. In fact, many patients ski and perform cheerleading activities while wearing their braces. When the brace is worn under clothing, it is not at all displeasing cosmetically, and with new advances in brace materials and proper selection of clothes, many patients tell me that their friends and acquaintances often forget that they are wearing braces. The brace can be removed for brief periods to allow for skin care and bathing. Scoliosis and kyphosis can be corrected simultaneously in the Milwaukee brace, and kyphotic deformities —especially from Scheuermann's disease—are receptive to Milwaukee brace correction (Fig. 10-3).

Techniques

When the Milwaukee brace was originally designed, a chin pad or rest was used that occasionally caused unsightly bite deformities. However, for the last 6 years a plastic throat mold designed by Blount has been used approximately

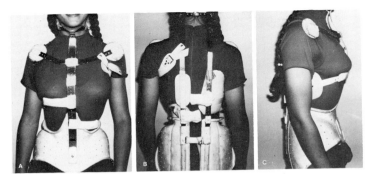

Fig. 10-3.   Well-made brace on a patient with scoliosis and kyphosis. Pelvic girdle fits perfectly and extends down to include buttocks on both sides. Lumbar lordosis has been completely corrected, and shoulders are held back by shoulder outriggers in front. Scoliosis is corrected with right thoracic L pad (*B* and *C*), and kyphotic deformity is corrected by posterior uprights and kyphosis pad seen in *B* on left posterior upright.

three fingerbreadths below the manidible, and the spectre of bite deformities no longer exists. The throat mold does not distract the mandible, but gently keeps the occiput centered over the occipital pads, which must be properly contoured to the occipital area on both sides (Fig. 10-4).

The adjustable thoracic and lumbar pads are best placed and observed with radiographic control over the ribs that lead to the apex of the curve in the thoracic region. A frequent mistake is to place the pressure pad directly over the apex of a curve, which then exerts an influence higher than desired. In the lumbar region, the lumbar pad must be placed low enough so that it is not striking any ribs or it will counteract the effect of the thoracic pad on the opposite side and tend to increase the thoracic curve.

Indications for The Milwaukee Brace

The Milwaukee brace is indicated for infantile and juvenile patients who have progressive curves but who are too young for operative intervention. Even some forms of congenital scoliosis can be held in this manner, but if curve progression in a young patient with congenital scoliosis is evident, these cases should be fused *in situ* without further delay. However, it is surprising how many years of extra spinal growth can be obtained by judicious Milwaukee bracing in selected congenital curves.

Secondly, the Milwaukee brace is most effective in the management of patients who are inoperable because of their general physical condition or a specifc type of terminal disease, such as muscular dystrophy or malignancy. The Milwaukee brace allows many of these patients to have practically normal spinal growth, and a more comfortable life can be obtained without the

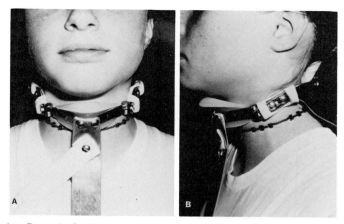

Fig. 10-4.   Properly fitted throat mold and occipital pads. Throat mold doesn't press against mandible but exerts slight pressure in front of throat, causing occiput to touch occipital pads that are slanted obliquely to fit at base of occiput on both sides. Neck ring should never constrict patient's throat or cause choking sensation in standing or sitting positions.

grotesque deformities that used to occur in the years before proper bracing.

The Milwaukee brace is most effective in treating patients with idiopathic scoliosis and most forms of roundback. During periods of adolescent growth most curves tend to become severe, and judicious bracing can halt further progression and actually improve many of these curves and hold them so that progression in adult life is minimal. A curve that originally is seen at 30° in a 14-year-old and is reduced to 15° by age 18 has much less chance of progressing in adult life—if the spine is in good balance—than a curve that is 30° at full maturity and is out of balance. Probably the ''ideal'' adolescent brace patient is a skeletally aged 15-year-old girl with a 35° thoracic or double major scoliosis who is cooperative and willing to wear the brace for 2 to 3 years. She will probably end up with a curve of 15° to 18° and should hold most of her correction through adult life. Curves such as this would almost certainly progress to surgery if not properly braced.

Constructing and Fitting the Milwaukee Brace

When the Milwaukee brace is applied, it must be worn 23 hours a day. This is a difficult period for the patient, but if the family is cooperative and the patient is not pampered too much, most patients learn to wear the brace 23 hours a day within 1 or 2 weeks of the initial application. The Milwaukee brace is constructed by the orthotist from a plaster pelvic impression that is custom made for each patient. Some scoliosis centers have started making ''stock'' pelvic corsets, which come in many standard sizes. These are less expensive and quite effective but do not have the exacting fit of a custom-made pelvic girdle, which usually provides better curve correction.

After the plaster impression has been taken, a positive mandril is made and the leather or plastic pelvic girdle molded to this form. In the past 2 years, polypropylene and polyethylene have been used with increasing success in our scoliosis clinic. These materials are lighter and more resistant to cracking and wear than previously used materials.

When the orthotist has finished the brace, the patient is fitted and all questions answered. It is important for the patient to be taught how to put the brace on and take it off since at first this seems to be a formidable process; however, it becomes extremely easy with practice.

The patient is then seen approximately 2 weeks after the initial fitting, at which time most straps and pads are adjusted to provide a proper fit. An x-ray taken at this time both in and out of the brace shows exactly where the pads are placed and if they are at the optimal locations for curve correction.

Subsequently, patients are seen at 3-month intervals and x-rays are taken both in and out of the brace at every second visit, or twice a year. As the patient matures, a single standing x-ray out of the brace is taken every 4 months to aid in the weaning process.

Timing of Treatment

When is a Milwaukee brace prescribed? When a young scoliotic patient is first seen and the curve is approximately 10° to 15°, I usually record all measurements and ask to see the patient again in 3 or 4 months with new films. As previously mentioned, some curves resolve spontaneously and stay permanently corrected. If these patients were to have been braced at the initial office visit, many of them would have been overtreated.

However, if significant curve progression has been shown on the second visit, Milwaukee bracing is promptly instituted. By significant progression I mean at least a 3° or 4° increase in the curve over a 3-month period.

Malignant curves progress rapidly in a short time. Parents are always warned against this and are told that if they notice a rapid increase in the size of the patient's rib deformity, they should come in for a much earlier appointment. If on subsequent visits a patient's curve does not progress or only changes 1° or 2°, a Milwaukee brace will not be prescribed, as long as a curve is under 20°. These patients often can be prevented from wearing a brace for 1 to 2 years before it is actually required. Once the brace is applied, it must be maintained until the patient is fully mature, which is usually about 18 years of age in girls and at least 12 or 18 months longer in boys.

Weaning

Milwaukee brace acceptance is usually good in adolescents 12 or 13 years of age. It is not until they reach 15 or 16 that social pressures increase and make brace wear less desirable. However, by this time the patient can usually begin to have some time out of the brace and the weaning process can be started. There is such a wide variety of individual response to the Milwaukee brace that it is difficult to state categorically how patients should be managed. Nevertheless, most patients will be held for 23 hours a day, and signs of secondary growth center formation—such as the vertebral ring apophyses and iliac crests—along with all the secondary growth characteristics previously mentioned should be closely observed.

Always remember to treat the patient and not the x-ray. Even though an x-ray may show good bony maturation, the major factor in determining whether more time out of the brace is advisable is maintenance of correction during the previous 3 months of a weaning attempt. For example, if a patient is out of the brace for 4 hours and has been holding her correction well for the previous 3 months, 6 hours of weaning per day can be tried. If in 3 more months new standing x-rays show maintenance of correction, another 2 hours out of the brace can be added. However, if the patient has lost several degrees during the past 3 months, the weaning time should be reduced or held at the present rate—no matter how skeletally mature the patient's x-rays may appear.

If a 15-year-old patient who has been in the brace for 18 months shows signs of maturation, an extra hour out of the brace can be allowed, which usually gives her 2 hours of freedom. This must be done only with the understanding that if the curve is more severe on the next x-ray examination, the patient will have to go back into the brace 23 hours a day. If this early attempt at weaning is successful, and no loss of correction occurs, the patient can be given another hour 3 months later.

The greatest mistake I made during my early enthusiastic years with the Milwaukee brace was to try to wean patients too early and too quickly. I am always sympathetic with these adolescents, but it is much better to obtain a proper scientific goal than to allow one's emotions to overrule sound medical judgment. The worst thing to do is to try to wean the patient out of the brace before the spine is ready, since then the curve almost certainly will progress and the patient will feel that the past 2 or 3 years in the brace have been wasted. If the weaning process is carried out slowly over several years, the results are much more satisfactory and a happy end result can be anticipated.

Even when the patient is in the brace for 23 hours a day, I usually allow them an extra hour a day for swimming during the summer and during winter vacations, as long as that time is spent immersed in the water or supine at poolside or a beach. Sitting without the brace is just as harmful as standing, and these activities should be discouraged since they will cause an increase in the curve if the patient's spine is too immature to allow them.

When the weaning process is started, it is important to encourage the patient and emphasize that you are not assuming God's role but are merely managing a medical condition to the best of your scientific ability. If the patient and family are convinced of this and realize that the effort must be a ''team'' one, which requires their help, the entire bracing experience will be much more successful for all concerned.

When I initially prescribe a brace for a young girl I am always asked, ''How long will I need to wear it?'' Never give the patient a specific time because if this goal is not realized, the patient will become despondent. Always tell the patient the truth. I usually answer that the brace will be needed until full maturity, but that I am as anxious to end treatment as the patient is and will do everything possible to get the best result in the shortest time. I point out that nature does not have a specific time clock and cannot be hurried. If the patient and family are totally unable to accept the time that bracing will require, surgery may be the best answer.

Evaluation of Milwaukee Brace Treatment

In 1970 Moe and Kettleson, evaluated 288 major idiopathic curves in 169 patients who had completed Milwaukee brace treatment or were wearing the brace at night only during the weaning process. The data collected and analyzed included the history, initial and final physical findings, roentgenograms of the spinal deformity, and the curves as determined at different evaluation times during and after treatment. These investigators concluded that: (1) major curves occurred in three distinct areas—high thoracic (from the seventh cervical vertebra to the seventh thoracic vertebra, thoracic (third thoracic to the third lumbar vertebra), and lumbar (tenth thoracic to the fifth lumbar vertebra; (2) median total brace wearing time was 34.3 months; (3) the best correction was obtained within the first 25 months in 97 percent of patients and within 2½ years in all patients; (4) high thoracic curves gave the poorest response, and thoracic and lumbar curves the best; (5) median loss for correction after removal of the brace was 1 percent in thoracic curves and 5 percent in lumbar curves; (6) the best response to brace treatment occurred when treatment was begun before the iliac epiphyses were closed and capped; (7) longer curves were corrected better than shorter curves; (8) only one curve of less than 40° at the start of brace treatment was surgically corrected, and this was an uncooperative patient; (9) certain small curves treated in the Milwaukee brace showed little or no final correction but were classified as satisfactory because the curves were not allowed to progress; (10) some larger double major curves of 45° to 50° of the right thoracic–left lumbar variety showed little x-ray improvement but still demonstrated substantial cosmetic results with better balance and lessening of the rib prominence (improvement produced by the brace was not necessarily quantitatively demonstrable); (11) marked deformities in some young patients were kept from progressing or even improved so that surgery could be safely delayed until a more desirable age for operation was reached; (12) the best results were obtained in patients and families who cooperated fully (Fig. 10-5).

The main advantages of the Milwaukee brace are that it prevents curve increase in a great percentage of patients, lessens the magnitude of the curve, improves body alignment, involves few risks, does not scar the skin, and leaves the spine fully mobile. The disadvantages of the Milwaukee brace are that it offers less correction than surgery in curves over 40°, there is less guarantee of a permanent result, the duration of treatment is considerably longer than surgical treatment, there are occasional psychological problems with prolonged brace wear, more frequent medical visits are necessary over a protracted period of time, and more x-ray exposure is required during this period.

Contraindications to Milwaukee brace treatment are thoracic lordosis, markedly decreased pulmonary function, a severe rib hump, a rigid scoliotic curve, an uncooperative patient, nonsupportive parents, the absence of a competent orthopedist or orthotist, geographical barriers, and socioeconomic-ethnic barriers.

Brace Prescriptions

What are the prescriptions to be ordered for the major types of scoliotic curves seen? We will start with the double major curve, which is almost always a right thoracic–left lumbar scoliosis. The proper brace prescription should read: (1) right thoracic 'L' pad (pad centered over ribs leading to apex of curve); (2) left lumbar pad; (3) left axillary sling.

This prescription allows effective correction of both curves and usually results in a rather rapid increase in the patient's body height; especially if both curves are over 25° (Fig. 10-6). The brace will require frequent adjustments, as maximum curve correction occurs during the first 6 to 9 months.

The next prescription is for a right thoracic curve, with a minimal left lumbar compensatory curve. In this case, one needs a Milwaukee brace with (1) a right thoracic 'L' pad, and (2) a left axillary sling.

A left lumbar pad need not be added initially because the basic premise here is to break the right thoracic curve into two components by actually increasing the left lumbar curve, creating two curves in proper balance. In effect, therefore, it is better to have two curves of 30° each in opposite directions with a well-balanced spine than to have a right thoracic curve of 40° and a left lumbar curve of 20° with the spine out of balance to the right.

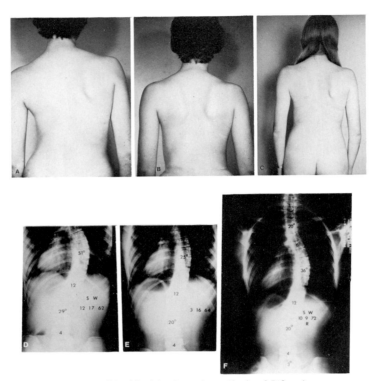

Fig. 10-5A   Adolescent girl with right thoracic scoliosis of 51° and compensatory left lumbar curve of 29°. (A and D were taken in December 1962.) Patient was placed in Milwaukee brace even though she was 16 years, 10 months of age because she was skeletally 1½ yrs. younger. In March 1964 correction was dramatic both cosmetically (B) and on x-rays (E), with reduction of thoracic curve from 51° to 25° and lumbar curve from 29° to 20° in erect position. Patient was then out of Milwaukee brace most of the time and returned for 8-year follow-up in October 1972, at age 25. C. She was maintaining a good cosmetic and functional correction. F. X-ray showed that curve had increased slightly to 36° in right thoracic, with 20° left high thoracic and left lumbar compensatory curves. She was a fully mature woman with no symptoms and spine in excellent balance. Chances of curve progressing in later life are slim; however, it she had not been treated in 1962, 51° curve would have become extremely severe when she was in her mid-30's. (Courtesy Walter P. Blount, M.D.)

Therefore we first apply only the thoracic 'L' pad on the right side and allow the lumbar curve to increase slightly until the thoracic curve has been reduced somewhat, at which time a left lumbar pad can be added. The axillary sling is usually applied on the side opposite the thoracic 'L' pad, and its main function is to keep the neck ring of the Milwaukee brace from digging into the neck on the opposite side of the thoracic pad. The axillary sling should never be tight

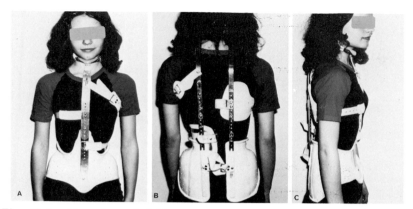

Fig. 10-6.   Properly made Milwaukee brace for double major scoliosis—right thoracic–left lumbar curve. *C*. Lumbar lordosis has been completely reduced, and neck ring comes about 2 fingerbreadths below mandible. Bodysuit fits patient snugly and does not allow wrinkles to develop between skin and pelvic girdle. Suits can be changed during day in hot weather so that skin does not macerate.

enough to cause occlusive vascular or neural problems and should be adjusted to the comfort of the patient and to center the neck ring.

Thoracolumbar curves are best managed by: (1) a low thoracic 'L' pad directly over the ribs leading to the apex of the curve, and (2) an axillary sling on the opposite side.

A lumbar pad is not used in treating these curves, since it would counteract the corrective effect of the thoracic pad. The prescription for a right thoracolumbar curve is: (1) a right thoracolumbar 'L' pad—low, and (2) a left axillary sling.

The last most common curve pattern is the lumbar curve, and for these a lumbar pad is always used as low as possible inside the pelvic girdle, but directly above the iliac crest so that maximum effect can be obtained and directed toward the lumbar spine. This pad should not touch the tips of the lower ribs, since it usually will then start to cause an increase in the compensatory curve above. Nevertheless, a slight increase may be desirable because again the goal is to break a major lumbar curve into two more acceptable curves; namely, thoracic and lumbar curves of opposite and nearly equal degrees. An axillary sling is usually added to the opposite side of the lumbar pad. The prescription for a left lumbar curve includes: (1) a left lumbar pad, and (2) a right axillary sling.

In patients with double major curves in the thoracic region, usually a left high thoracic–right low thoracic curve, the left shoulder is much higher than the right, and the entire shoulder girdle must be pulled down and inward to effect proper cosmetic improvement and curve reduction. This is generally best done with a device called a ring flange, although a single half-ring of thermoplastic material (a "trapezius" pad) can be placed directly over the trapezius muscle down to the uprights of the brace to effect proper correction. A thoracic 'L' pad then must be used over the lower thoracic curve directly against the ribs leading to the apex of that curve (Fig. 10-7). Sometimes as these curves are corrected, a left lumbar pad has to be used over the compensatory lumbar curve that often develops.

The prescription for a left high thoracic–low right thoracic curve should read: (1) left shoulder trapezius pad (or ring flange), and (2) right thoracic 'L' pad.

An important thing to remember about all treatment with the Milwaukee brace is that these curves are always dynamic. That is, they are ever changing, and a specific Milwaukee brace prescription may have to be changed and pads placed from right to left depending on what happens to the major and compensatory curves being treated. Several patients have had total reversal of curves, especially in the thoracolumbar region, and careful management is necessary with adequate x-ray control in the brace to be certain that curves are not being overcorrected or that other curves are being created in opposite directions (Fig. 10-8). That is why in the first 18 months of brace wear, especially in children 10 to 14 years old, x-rays are always taken in and out of the brace at 6-month intervals. The basic technique of brace treatment is to divide and conquer. Attempt to reduce a major curve into two opposite but equal cosmetically and functionally acceptable curves; then hold them until full maturity.

Although the ideal brace patient is a fairly mature 15-year-old girl with a 25° to 30° scoliosis, the brace many times needs to be used in patients 9 and 10 years old. I feel that it is much more conservative to manage such juvenile patients in the Milwaukee brace until they are old enough for surgical intervention, usually around age 14. The patient thus has had beneficial effects of judicious brace wear during periods of active development, but brace treatment can then be interrupted for rapid surgical correction and termination of all scoliosis treatment 9 months after surgery. The interruption of prolonged brace treatment is an excellent indication for surgical intervention, and a combination of bracing and surgery is used most often in many patients.

If my 10-year-old daughter had advancing scoliosis, I would wish to have her braced for 3 or 4 years and then undergo surgery by a skilled technician. This way she would have the best treatment and still have a relatively fully grown spine at the time of surgery, with the knowledge that she would have an excellent correction and be freed of all bracing and casting by the time she was 15.

There is no single perfect treatment for scoliosis. Scoliosis management must consist of a combination of bracing, casting, and surgery in many instances to effect a proper end result. Unfortunately, bracing is sometimes

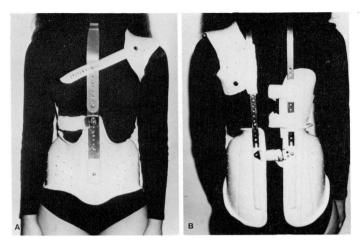

Fig. 10-7.   Properly made Milwaukee brace for double thoracic scoliosis—high left thoracic curve and low right thoracic scoliosis. Shoulder ring flange on left pulls high left shoulder down and in. Right lower thoracic L pad is centered over tips of ribs leading to apex of scoliosis on right. A new modification for pulling down high-riding upper thoracic curve and shoulder is trapezius pad, which does not go under arm but gently effects pressure over trapezius muscle mass and is anchored to uprights in front and back of brace to pull shoulder down. These high thoracic curves are difficult to manage because of presence of arm and shoulder and inability to affect direct rib pressure in axillary region.

considered conservative and surgery radical. A person with a ruptured appendix who has nonoperative treatment is certainly not receiving conservative care, but is being treated radically and will most likely die of ensuing peritonitis. In this patient, a surgical approach would be the conservative treatment. This is likewise true in scoliotic patients, and sound judgment must be exercised, depending on the attitudes of the patient and parents.

Many of my patients have rejected Milwaukee bracing and have practically insisted on surgical management right from the onset for curves that may have responded well to the brace. On the other hand, other families and patients have rejected any thought or suggestion of surgery, even in cases of advanced curves of 60° or 70°. The proper advice and treatment for patients must be individualized and no specific rules can be followed.

Milwaukee Brace Exercises

Proper Milwaukee brace exercises, both in and out of the brace, have been defined and illustrated by Blount and Moe in their excellent text on the Milwaukee brace. The exercises to be done outside of the Milwaukee brace are generally held to a count of 5 and done 10 times each. The exercises include: (1)

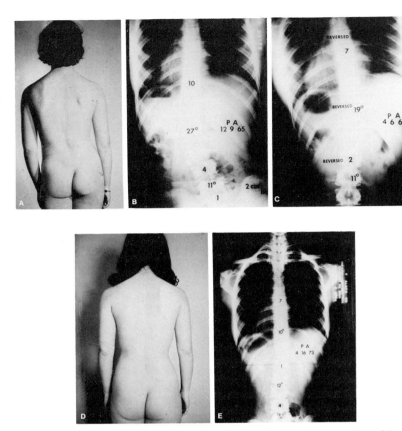

Fig. 10-8*A*.   Adolescent girl first seen in 1965 with leg length shortening of 2 cm on left side. Since her bone age and chronologic age were exactly 13, right distal femoral epiphyseal closure was performed at that time. This corrected pelvic obliquity over next several years as leg length discrepancy decreased. Patient was placed in a Milwaukee brace, scoliotic curves reversed from original left thoracolumbar curve of 27° to 19° in opposite direction. She was extremely supple for her age. In April 1973 (*D* and *E*) she was 21 years old and correction was holding perfectly. Spine was in balance, and cosmetic and functional end result was excellent. (Courtesy Walter P. Blount, M.D.)

pelvic tilt, supine, with the knees flexed; (2) pelvic tilt, with knees straight; (3) sit-ups, with pelvic tilt held; (4) pelvic tilt in the standing position; (5) upper, middle, and lower thorax breathing exercises; (6) spine extension in the prone position; (7) push-ups, with pelvis tilted.

Exercises to be done in the Milwaukee brace should be done to the count of 5 and generally are done 10 times daily. (The last two exercises can be done many times a day.) They include: (1) pelvic tilt, supine, with knees flexed; (2)

pelvic tilt, supine, with knees straight; (3) pelvic tilt, standing; (4) spine extension in the prone position; (5) push-ups with the pelvis tilted; (6) correction of the thoracic lordosis and rib hump; (7) active correction of the major curve by tilting the pelvis and shifting the torso away from the thoracic pad.

These exercises are most effective when done every day and should be supervised at least at biweekly intervals when the brace is first applied and subsequently at monthly visits to the physiotherapist.

OTHER BRACES FOR SCOLIOSIS

During the past several years, others have attempted scoliosis bracing using different types of thermoplastic material, as well as braces that do not extend up to the neck. This is perhaps the main objection to the Milwaukee brace and the cause of most patient rejection. Adolescents are so sensitive about appearance that a small pimple can seem to be the size of a basketball. Likewise, they feel that everyone notices their Milwaukee brace and that it is really much more unsightly than it actually is.

For these reasons, clinics throughout the United States and other parts of the world have been attempting to develop braces that will not require extensions up to and including the neck. Some of these molded corsets and braces are effective, especially in thoracolumbar and lumbar curves (Fig. 10-9).

Under the direction of Dr. David B. Levine, the Prenyl brace has been used successfully at the Hospital for Special Surgery. The polypropylene brace with a soft Allomed lining is being prefabricated in several pelvic sizes under the direction of Dr. John E. Hall in Boston with encouraging early results. Finally, thermoplastic body jackets, originally described by Cockrell and Risser, have been recently incorporated into our brace regimen for managing thoracolumbar and lumbar deformities (Fig. 10-10).

All three forms of body jackets have advantages and disadvantages, but it is still too early to determine the exact placement of each type of material and technique in the treatment of scoliotic patients. Excellent spinal management can be obtained by all of these braces if the patient is not severely concerned about cosmesis and is willing to wear the appliance for the proper length of time to ensure adequate treatment.

In France, many patients have been treated over the last few years with the Lyonnaise brace, which is an underarm brace with a holding pad at the apex of a lumbar or thoracolumbar curve. A similar brace is also used by Ponti in Italy; both of these braces appear to be effective for flexible mild lumbar and thoracolumbar curves. They are usually not satisfactory for thoracic or double major curve patterns.

The decision for the proper treatment of scoliosis in curves of 20° to 25° is

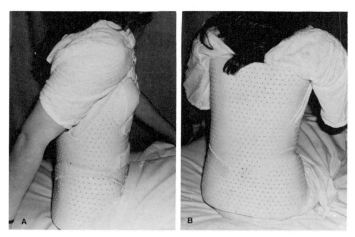

Fig. 10-9.   Orthoplast girdle constructed for paraplegic with kyphotic deformity. She was extremely supple and tolerated this form of spinal support quite well, which allowed her to sit erect and use her wheelchair more effectively.

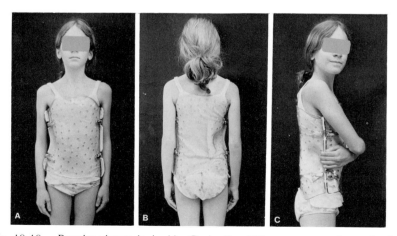

Fig. 10-10.   Pasadena brace devised by Cockrell and Risser to correct thoracolumbar and lumbar curves without need for extending brace above shoulders. This form of bracing is effective for lower curves, and as curve correction continues, more pressure is made over inverted pressure pad at apex of curve with subsequent braces. Like Milwaukee brace, Pasadena brace can be constructed only by a properly trained orthotist.

156

generally quite easy. Most of these patients, especially adolescents, should have Milwaukee bracing. Likewise, it is generally easy to make the proper decision for patients with curves of 45° to 60°, because most of these patients should have a surgical approach. The difficult area is what we refer to as the "grey zone," between 35° and 50°; many of these patients may respond to proper bracing, but psychologically they may do better with the surgical approach. Therefore, each case must be evaluated depending upon the patient's psychological acceptance of bracing, the flexibility of the curve, the patient's physical and emotional maturity, and the parents' sophistication and experience. Many cases considered "brace failures" really are patients who had braces applied at 50° or 60°; the failure was actually in proper treatment selection. These patients initially should have been treated surgically rather than being started on an almost certain course of failure with the brace.

Although the Milwaukee brace will remain the mainstay of scoliosis bracing and nonoperative treatment, experimental designs in a wide variety of new materials will continue to be carreid out to improve brace design, manufacutre, strength, weight, comfort, and durability. Available orthotic appliances properly made and worn can effectively treat many curvatures of the spine. Specific problems such as malignant scoliosis, neurofibromatosis, congenital kyphosis, and congenital hemivertebra, unilateral bars, and thoracic lordosis are specific contraindications to brace treatment and require spinal fusion. Most other scoliotic curves respond properly to brace care. The main objective of bracing should be to prevent small curves from becoming large curves. It is important, therefore, to start brace treatment promptly when the need is first recognized and to continue bracing until the problem has been solved by adequate curve correction or the obvious evidence that some other form of treatment has become necessary.

REFERENCES

1. Barash HL, DeWald R:Milwaukee brace treatment for idiopathic scoliosis. J Bone Joint Surg 53A:196, 1971
2. Blount WP,Moe JH: TheMilwaukee Brace. Baltimore, Williams & Wilkins, 1973
3. Blount WP: Scoliosis and theMilwaukee brace. Bull Hosp Joint Dis 19:152, 1958
4. Blount WP: Non-operative treatment of scoliosis. Symposium of the Spine, American Academy of Orthopaedic Surgeons, Cleveland, 1967. St. Louis, Mosby, 1969, p 188
5. Blount WP, Bolinske J: Physical therapy in the nonoperative treatment of scoliosis. Phys Ther Rev 47:919, 1967
6. Blount WP,Mellencamp DD: Scoliosis treatment—skeletal maturity evaluation. Minn Med 56:382, 1973
7. Blount WP, Schmidt AC, Keever D, et al: TheMilwaukee brace in the operative treatment of scoliosis. J Bone Joint Dis 40A:511, 1958

8. Bradford D, Moe JH, Winter RB: Adolescent kyphosis. Minn Med 56:114, 1973
9. Bradford D, Moe J, Winter R et al: Exhibit at the annual meeting of the American Academy of Orthopaedic Surgeons, Las Vegas, 1973
10. Cockrell R, Risser J: Plastic body jacket in the treatment of scoliosis. Exhibit at the annual meeting of the American Academy of Orthopaedic Surgeons, Las Vegas, 1973
11. Duval-Beaupere G: Pathogenic relationship between scoliosis and growth, in Zorab P: Scoliosis and Growth. London, Churchill-Livingstone, 1971, p 58
12. Edmondson AS, Morris JT: Analysis of a follow-up study of Milwaukee brace treatment in patients with idiopathic scoliosis. Presented to the Scoliosis Research Society, Wilmington, 1972
13. Greulich WW, Pyle SI: Radiographic Atlas of Skeletal Development of the Hand and Wrist. Stanford, Stanford University Press, 1966
14. James JIP: Infantile idiopathic scoliosis. Clin Orthop 77:57, 1971
15. Moe JH: Treatment of adolescent kyphosis by non-operative and operative methods. Manitoba Med Rev 8:45:481, 1965
16. Moe JH: The Milwaukee brace in the treatment of scoliosis. Clin Orthop 77:18, 1971
17. Moe JH, Kettelson DN: Analysis of curve pattern and preliminary results of Milwaukee brace treatment in 169 patients. J Bone Joint Surg 52A:1509, 1970
18. Myers BA, Friedman SB, Weiner IB: Coping with a chronic disability: psychosocial observations of girls with scoliosis treated with a Milwaukee brace. Dis Child 120:175, 1970
19. Paul SW: Five years of non-operative treatment of scoliosis and kyphosis: a follow-up study. Orthot Prosthet 22:28, 1968
20. Shufflebarger H, Keiser R: Results of Milwaukee brace treatment in idiopathic scoliosis. Personal communication.
21. Tanner JM: Some main features of normal growth in children, in Zorab P: Scoliosis and Growth. London, Churchill-Livingstone, 1971, p 23
22. Winter RB, Moe JH: Idiopathic scoliosis, current concepts in treatment. Minn Med 55:529, 1972
23. Winter RB, Moe JH, Eilers, VE: Congenital scoliosis: a study of 234 patients treated and untreated. J Bone Joint Surg 50A:1, 1968
24. Winter RB, Moe JH, Wang JF: Congenital kyphosis. J Bone Joint Surg 55A:223, 1973
25. Winter RB, Moe JH: Orthotics for spinal deformity. Clin Orthop 102:72–91, 1974

11

The Operative Management of Scoliosis

HISTORY

For centuries surgeons have been looking for better methods. Spinal surgery has always been considered one of the most difficult and demanding forms of surgery. The first spine fusion was performed in 1911 by Hibbs at the old New York Orthopaedic Hospital. The patient had tuberculosis, and a posterior fusion operation was performed to immobilize the spine and control the disease process.

Hibbs' techniques worked so well that his fame quickly spread and inspired the medical community. He established new standards of surgical excellence that have stood the test of time and are still being used at the New York Orthopaedic Hospital of the Columbia-Presbyterian Medical Center.

Then in 1914 Hibbs performed the first scoliosis spine fusion. He reasoned that the curvature could be arrested by fusing the vertebrae to each other, the same as if one were trying to weld the links of a chain to immobilize it. Hibbs' courage in exploring new surgical horizons is even more surprising when one considers that his work was done many decades before blood transfusions, antibiotics, and anesthetic techniques became available to make this type of surgery less hazardous.

Hibbs' discovery of the spinal fusion rapidly spread among his colleagues, and within the next 10 years many surgeons skillfully attempted to improve on his techniques. Many new methods were devised, and our present surgical endeavors are a distillation of the expertise of our forefathers. As blood typing and transfusions became possible and anesthetic techniques improved, longer and longer spine fusions were performed in one sitting.

Until about 10 years ago, however, it was customary to fuse no more than three or four vertebrae in one sitting and to stage the procedures so that a 12- or 13-vertebrae scoliosis fusion would be done in three stages over a 3- or 4-month period. The patients would be placed in corrective plaster casts after surgery and would be held from 9 to 12 months in the supine position with various dynamic casting techniques to correct the deformed spine.

Among Hibbs' disciples were Risser and Von Lackum, who added procedures of their own to establish better fusion and cast methods for treating patients with spinal deformities. Risser established the localizer cast technique in New York. Because of ill health, he moved early in his career to California, where he continued to establish a worldwide reputation of excellence in spinal correction using the localizer cast and spinal fusion with local bone graft. Von Lackum remained at the New York Orthopaedic Hospital and devised the surcingle cast technique and a method of spine fusion with early ambulation that resulted in excellent corrections and long-lasting results. His patients are still seen regularly in our follow-up clinics.

While Risser and Von Lackum were experimenting, Moe and Goldstein perfected fusion techniques consisting of individual facet fusion; Moe originally described this technique for treating scoliosis, especially in the thoracic and lumbar regions. Goldstein added to our knowledge of fusion techniques by his total decortication procedure, in which the entire laminar areas and all facet joints are totally denuded of cortical bone, and large amounts of autogenous cancellous and cortical bony strips are interlaced throughout the area to be fused, promoting sound and permanent spinal fusion. Cobb devised an x-ray measurement technique used daily throughout the world that has contributed greatly to our understanding of the pathogenesis of scoliosis.

During the early 1940s, Harrington developed posterior instruments, which consisted of a distraction rod placed on the concave side of a curve, and a compression device applied to the convex side for the dynamic correction of scoliosis during surgery. At first, Harrington envisioned his technique to be used without spinal fusion and without plaster. He believed that it was possible to correct the spine and then remove the instruments when full growth was achieved, thereby leaving the patient with mobile spinal segments. However, it soon became obvious that the metal instruments would cut out of bone unless a spine fusion was performed at the same time as instrumentation. Harrington continued to experiment with dozens of different hooks, rods, and insertion techniques until he discovered the right combination of Harrington distraction and compression assemblies and a ''dowel'' technique for bone grafting using cylindrical plugs cut from the iliac crest. These plugs were then inserted into the facet joints, especially in the thoracic and thoracolumbar regions. Harrington instrumentation has been the most significant advancement in treating spinal deformities in the last 30 years.

During the 1950s and 1960s, Hodgson devised anterior spinal fusion techniques for evacuating tuberculous abscesses and used rib strut grafts for fusion material. His surgical approaches and techniques inspired Dwyer of Australia to devise a cable-bolt system for the anterior correction of spinal deformities from the convex side. Dwyer's technique has evolved over the last 15 years and has been extremely dramatic for specific types of curve correction, especially in patients with previously unsuccessful posterior spinal surgery or patients with missing posterior elements, such as meningomyelocele, where an anterior fusion is the only reasonable approach.

Over the last 20 years, techniques have made scoliosis spinal surgery safer, more effective, and permanently rewarding, with lasting correction in the vast majority of patients. Nevertheless, there is no question that operative treatment over the last 20 years has become safer and more effective; however, we must guard against the possibility of spinal surgery becoming more dangerous. This paradox is possible because our techniques for corrective surgery are now becoming so powerful and our methods of spinal control are so great through instrumentation and plaster techniques that the chances of surgically over-stretching anatomical structures are increasing. Most (85 percent) of our patients requiring surgery have simple, uncomplicated problems that can easily be managed by routine correction and spine fusion. Complications occur mainly in the 15 percent of the more difficult cases that involve neurological deficits and other metabolic and physical problems leading to more hazardous and complicated spinal surgery.

There are several primary indications for surgical treatment of spinal deformities: (1) progression of the deformity, especially in congenital scoliosis; (2) pain; (3) progressive respiratory deficit (noted specifically in curves over 60° by Cobb measurement; (4) neurological impairment; (5) prevention of future problems such as degenerative arthritic changes and destruction of facet joints; (6) cosmesis, which is becoming more important as our society becomes more sophisticated; (7) sitting stability, which is extremely important in patients with neurological and congenital spinal problems who need a stable spine to propel themselves in wheelchairs or other devices.

Progressive deformity is becoming an increasingly severe physical and psychological problem. I often see families in which the parents or the child will not tolerate a curve over 25° or 30°. The parents are most insistent that their child's back be absolutely straight, and although some parents are unreasonable in this regard, deformities that were socially acceptable years ago are no longer generally tolerated by our society.

Most scoliotic curves over 45° should be treated surgically, especially if the spine is out of balance. Curves in that range often can be successfully braced, but the attitudes of the parents and patient must be carefully assessed. Some of my patients will not tolerate a curve over 35° and are extremely anxious to have correction performed as quickly as possible. Psychologically, they are opposed to wearing any type of brace for a long time and they readily respond to the suggestion of surgery. It is not the surgeon's role to force a specific treatment on a patient. Two young girls with identical curves may undergo different forms of treatment because one may accept 3 or 4 years of daily spinal bracing, whereas the other may reject bracing in favor of surgery, which generally results in a straight, stable, and permanently corrected spine 9 months after treatment.

I believe that the correction of a 40° scoliosis in an otherwise healthy 14-year-old patient when performed in a modern hospital setting with good anesthesia, surgical technique, and blood banking, is no more dangerous than driving from New York City to Florida or California. Adult scoliotic patients are being operated on with greater frequency now that surgical and anesthetic techniques have been improved so greatly. Nevertheless, adults have more postoperative complications and psychological difficulties than adolescents. It is unfortunate to see the number of adults who could have undergone surgery as adolescents and later have to endure much more hardship and obtain less correction because their spines are more rigid (Fig. 11-1).

Progressive congenital scoliosis requires surgical treatment because brace treatment is almost always inadequate for congenital curves. Most congenital curves should be fused in situ as soon as progression is noted.

Paralytic curves almost always need surgical treatment because even after full maturity, the paralytic components that contributed to the patient's scoliosis continue and these curves become extremely severe if nothing is done to halt their progression. Fortunately, we see fewer patients with paralysis from polio all the time; however, myelomeningocele, cerebral palsy, progressive spinal atrophy, and traumatic paraplegic patients should undergo prompt surgical fusion to stabilize their spines. In patients with diseases known to cause severe scoliosis, especially such conditions as neurofibromatosis, the spine should be fused without hesitation.

Pain is becoming a more commonly accepted indication for surgical intervention. Pain is so subjective that it varies with the patient's background, education, religion, and ethnic group. However, many psychologically stable people have unrelenting pain that is unresponsive to all forms of conservative treatment. When this pain is located in the curve and the other possibilities for pain production have been eliminated, surgical stabilization should be considered, especially in adults. Most adolescents have no symptoms, but the presence of symptoms in a maturing teen-ager or young adult is certainly indicative of greater pain in the future (Fig. 11-2).

The third indication for surgery is increasing respiratory deficit. This entity has been so thoroughly documented by pulmonary function studies in the past 30 years that there is little doubt that patients with scoliosis over 50° or 60°

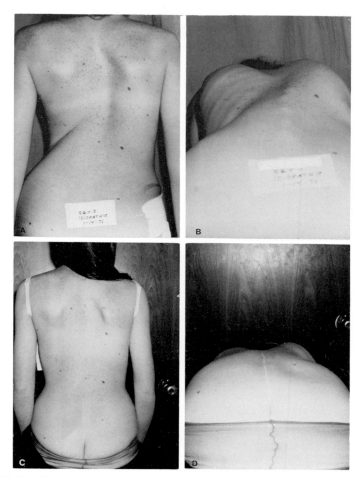

Fig. 11-1. 22-year-old girl first seen in 1971 who had been followed for previous 6 years and told that scoliosis would never progress. At age 16 she had 48° right thoracic curve, and at this time presented with 105° right thoracic curve. Deformity caused severe psychological problems and increasing back pain and shortness of breath. *A*, *B*. She was placed in halofemoral traction, and after 10 days curve was reduced from 105° to 58° *(F)*. Then surgical correction reduced curve to 48°. She was held in halo cast for 9 months after surgery and was dramatically improved in all aspects. *C*, *D*. Patient in February 1975, at age 26 years, 4 months. She had become an airline stewardess, had recently married, and was extremely happy with her appearance. Curve maintained excellent, painless correction and measured 51° in right thoracic region *(G)*.

163

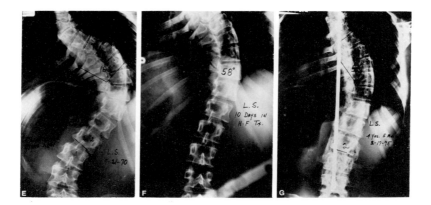

will have increasing cardiopulmonary difficulty leading to an early death (Fig. 11-3). Spinal stabilization increases the ventilation-perfusion ratio in the lungs and also prevents the curves from getting worse in the future, thereby adding years of life and comfort to the pulmonary cripple. Surgery, especially in severely deformed individuals, should be carefully done and is generally performed in stages since these patients have a low respiratory reserve and occasionally additional techniques, such as tracheostomy, are necessary.

The fourth indication for surgery is neurological involvement. The existence of nerve deficit or impending paraplegia in the lower extremities is an extremely grave and urgent indication for surgery. These patients many times respond to gentle traction techniques over a long period of time, such as 3 or 4 weeks, to allow the nerve roots and spinal cord to become decompressed. Without surgery and spinal stablization, usually combined with neural decompression, the prognosis for these patients is usually extremely grave. Occasionally only a spinal fusion is necessary, but in some instances a decompression of the entire neural canal, generally from an anterior approach, is required, along with anterior strut grafting and posterior spinal fusion.

The fifth indication for surgery is prevention of future degenerative problems in the spine. Our long follow-up studies illustrate what happens to a patient's spine when it is out of balance. Most adult patients with scoliosis develop respiratory, neurologic, or arthritic conditions that lead to increasing disability and pain. Many 20-year-old patients with 60° scoliotic curves are asymptomatic when first seen (Fig. 11-4). Yet as they grow older, these patients will have increasing deformity and severe disability. They should be promptly treated by surgical correction and fusion so that these problems are eliminated before they assume greater magnitude (Fig. 11-5). Unfortunately, for many years well-meaning physicians have told patients that their scoliotic curves will not progress after they are mature. This has been demonstrated numerous times

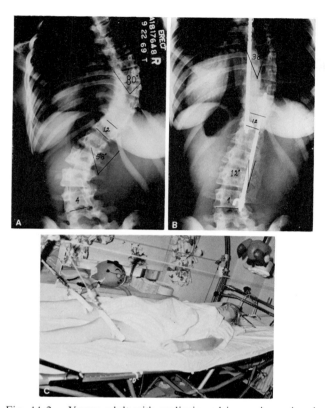

Fig. 11-2.   Young adult with scoliosis and increasing pain who
was first seen at age 16 years, 9 months. Surgical correction for 75°
right thoracic curve and 50° left lumbar scoliosis was advised.
Family at first refused, but agreed due to increasing pain when child
was 18½. At admission *(A)*, right thoracic scoliosis was 80° and left
lumbar curve 58° . She was placed in halofemoral traction *(C)* for 3
weeks preoperatively, and 2 Harrington rods were overlapped to
correct double major curves. This type of rod placement is extremely effective, but should be used with caution, especially in
severe curves, because spine is actually lengthened several cm, and
neurological damage is possible. *B.* Thoracic curve reduced to 38°
and lumbar curve to 12°.

to be untrue, and continuing disabling deformities have been allowed to
progress unchecked into adult life. By the time a middle-aged patient arrives
with severe pain and neurologic deficit, it is often too late to correct the situation
adequately.

The sixth surgical indication is cosmesis. Orthopedic surgeons are fre-

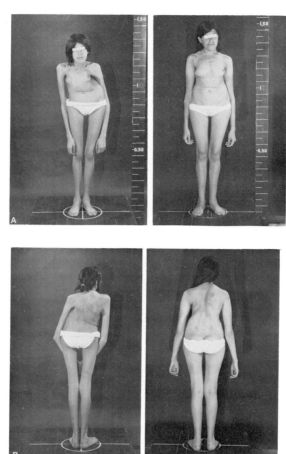

Fig. 11-3.   Adolescent girl who had severe kyphoscoliosis result-
ing in marked trunk shortening and respiratory deficit. She was
developing early neurologic problems with impending paraplegia.
Skeletal traction followed by scoliosis spinal surgery performed by
Cotrel produced this amazing end result. (Courtesy Professor
Yves Cotrel.)

quently criticized for performing scoliosis surgery on the basis that it is simply
cosmetic surgery. Although cosmesis should not be the major indication for
surgery, it certainly can be a pleasing by-product. Who is not concerned about
his appearance? Men and women spend millions of dollars annually to help
enhance their appearance and dress. What can be more psychologically and
physically disturbing to a patient, especially an adolescent girl, than an unsightly rib hump that is obvious to her friends, and even more so to her own

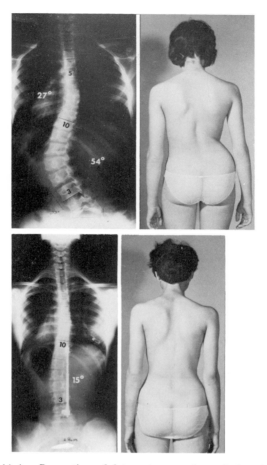

Fig. 11-4.   Prevention of future degenerative spinal problems.
Adolescent patient had 54° left lumbar curve with advanced rotational deformity. Spine was out of balance, which would cause
increasing low back pain in later life. Surgical correction with
Harrington instrumentation reduced curve to 15°. (Reprinted with
permission from Goldstein.[10])

psyche? Although I am primarily satisfied by knowing that surgery may have
prevented future curve progression and an early death, the most obvious source
of happiness for the patient and family is the fact that appearance has been
improved. Surgeons must not be chagrined by the fact that they are doing
cosmetic surgery, for they are also correcting deformity and preventing future
disability. Patient care at its best consists of treating the whole patient-
—physically and emotionally.

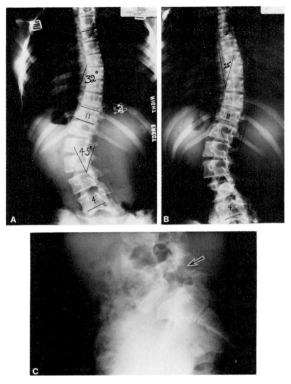

Fig. 11-5.   Prevention of future degenerative problems by combined surgical and brace treatment. 15-year-old girl, first seen in
1971 with right thoracic scoliosis of 32°, left lumbar curve of 45°,
and grade I spondylolisthesis, was already having hamstring tight-
ness in lower extremities. Fusion of spine to sacrum with resulting
limitation of motion was considered to be overwhelming treatment.
Although it was felt that she had independent spondylolisthesis as
well as idiopathic scoliosis, spondylolisthesis was fused from L-4 to
sacrum, and she was held in corrective scoliosis cast including 1 leg
to midthigh for 6 months. She was then placed in aMilwaukee brace
until she was 18, when cosmetic and functional results were excellent. She should have a normal adult life and has excellent spinal
mobility.

The final indication for surgery is spinal stability. With new techniques for rehabilitating paralyzed patients, we are much more cognizant of the importance of good sitting stability so that the patient has both arms and hands free to perform the activities of daily living, and also to manipulate a wheelchair and other mechanical devices. Spinal instability occurs in all paralytic problems, such as traumatic paraplegia, cerebral palsy, spinal muscular atrophy, polio, and muscular dystrophy. Pre- and postoperative films of patients with severe spinal paralysis who have undergone spinal arthrodesis illustrate how surgery improves these patients' ability to perform daily activities.

PLASTER TECHNIQUES

The discovery of plaster techniques by the Flemish military surgeon Antonius Mathysen in 1852 was a monumental step in the treatment of limb and spine deformities. Since that time, ingenious plaster techniques have been developed which, when coupled with proper corrective surgery, can correct even extremely resistant curves.

The original casting methods employed the turnbuckle cast, which Hibbs and Risser used at the New York Orthopaedic Hospital. A turnbucle was incorporated in sections of the cast, and a wedge was removed from the plaster itself. The turnbuckles were then opened on one side to close the removed plaster wedge with subsequent spinal correction. The turnbuckle cast, extremely popular during the 1930s and 1940s, provided effective, dynamic correction of recalcitrant paralytic curves. In fact, such great forces were exerted that severe pressure sores were often caused and spines were actually overcorrected.

Risser obtained the same dramatic corrections with his localizer plaster technique. This incorporated the principles of cephalopelvic traction in a longitudinal plane, while a pressure device called a localizer was applied directly over the apex of the major curve or curves. An actual plaster slab was pressed directly over the apex of the deformity and held in position while an incorporating plaster jacket was applied. The Risser technique has been extremely effective and is still practiced in most institutions with excellent results. During the last 20 years, Cotrel has devised the Cotrel sling technique. This provides spinal correction also using cephalopelvic traction and correcting slings, which are applied on the outside of the rapidly applied plaster as it is setting. The Cotrel technique is a dynamic and excellent method of correcting spinal deformities and is used throughout Europe and in some parts of this country (Figure 11-6).

As previously mentioned, Von Lackum originated the surcingle cast technique at the New York Orthopaedic Hospital during the 1930s and 1940s

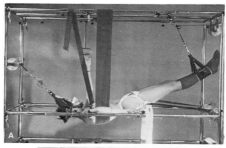

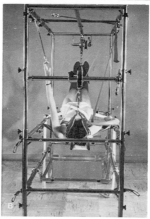

Fig. 11-6.   Cotrel technique for elongation, derotation, and flexion correction of scoliotic deformities. Patient is placed in cephalopelvic traction and derotation straps are applied to correct rib deformity on convex side during plaster application. These illustrations have been made on a model without plaster applied. Normally plaster is applied rapidly and straps are applied externally to the plaster while it is setting to correct structural deformities of ribs. (Courtesy Professor Yves Cotrel.)

(Fig. 11-7). The word ''surcingle'' was adapted from the training sling that is usually placed around the underbelly of a young horse during training. Surcingles can exert considerable pressure, and Von Lackum quickly perceived that such applied pressure could help the patient with spinal deformity. He first conceived of placing the patient face down on a wooden frame, pulling the patient on both sides directly over the apices of each curve, and holding these curves in the proper corrective position until the entire plaster jacket could be applied.

During the last 10 years of his life, Von Lackum devised a specific corrective casting and surgical technique that consisted of operating on the patient on his modernized surcingle-surgical frame. Then immediately after

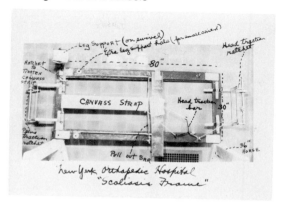

Fig. 11-7. Original Von Lackum surcingle frame made from
metal and wood at New York Orthopaedic Hospital in early 1930s.
Many excellent spinal corrections were obtained with this makeshift
scoliosis frame.

surgery, while the patient was still asleep, he applied a postoperative cast and
brought the patient to the recovery room on the frame. Then patient was held in
this cast for 9 months until bony union was complete. Most techniques used at
that time consisted of keeping the patient supine for at least 9 months, and many
surgeons during the 1930s and 1940s performed scoliosis surgery in stages 3 to
4 weeks apart.

Because I was originally trained to use the Risser localizer technique, I
was quite skeptical when first exposed to the Von Lackum surcingle method.
However, over the past 8 years I have realized that the surcingle technique
combines most of the advantages of all known plaster techniques, and, in
conjunction with a Cotrel frame, it can be used for the application of all types of
scoliosis and spinal casts (Fig. 11-8).

With the surcingle technique, the patient is held in the supine position with
the head in cephalopelvic distraction while lateral surcingle traction is applied
over the apex of each curve. The plaster is molded to the chin, occiput, and
pelvis during distraction. The surcingle straps exert their corrective forces
while the plaster is setting, and the plaster is applied in one layer from the head
to the pelvis, without joining separate individual sections as in other techniques. The rib deformity is greatly diminished in the thoracic region by the use
of the derotation principle of the thoracic surcingle strap (Fig. 11-9).

It is pointless to advocate one plaster technique over another, since the
technician's skill is so important. The technique a surgeon uses probably makes
little difference in the final outcome so long as he is an expert at applying
corrective traction forces and plaster. No matter how adequately performed the
surgery and how skillfully bone grafts are used, if the plaster technique does not
properly immobilize the spine in the corrected position for the prescribed
period of time, a permanent spinal deformity will remain.

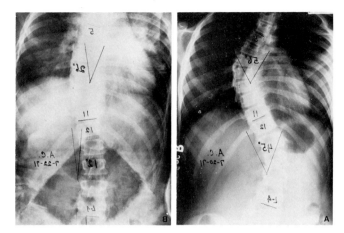

Fig. 11-8. Pre- and postoperative x-rays showing dramatic preoperative cast correction obtained using surcingle technique. Patient originally had 56° right thoracic scoliosis and 45° left lumbar curve. In 1 preoperative cast correction, curves were reduced to 26° and 12°, respectively. At surgery, further correction resulted in a practically straight spine. (Reprinted with permission, Keim HA, Waugh TR: The surcingle cast in scoliosis treatment. Clin Orthop 86:157, 1972.)

The important consideration in the treatment of scoliosis is not using metal implants or individually fusing facet joints. The basic surgical principles of clean dissection with ample decortication, adequate bone grafting using autogenous cancellous and cortical bone, and proper postoperative immobilization are the mainstays of corrective spinal surgery.

TRACTION METHODS

Halofemoral traction was first devised at Rancho los Amigos Hospital in the Los Angeles area. Garrett, Nickel, and Perry contributed greatly to corrective spinal techniques by adopting principles previously used in dental and maxillofacial surgery for applying cranial halofemoral pins for distraction over a long period of time. Halofemoral traction consists of inserting a cranial halo and heavy femoral pins, and using a turning frame 2 to 3 weeks preoperatively. Severely rigid and progressing spinal deformities can be slowly distracted and neurological complications avoided by adding weights slowly to the head and legs (Fig. 11-2C).

Halofemoral traction is extremely effective, especially in patients with paralytic deformities or fixed pelvic obliquities and rigid curves. Usually after 3

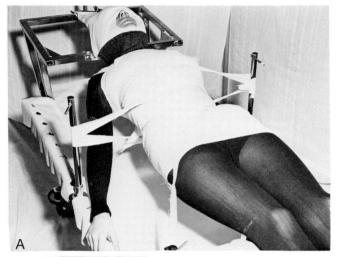

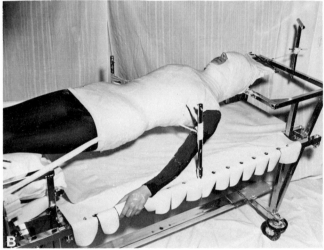

Fig. 11-9 *A*. Patient in cephalopelvic traction using disposable cervical halter around chin and occiput and criss-cross muslin straps over pelvis. Surcingle straps exert traction effect directly over apices of major curves, in this case right thoracic–left lumbar curve. *B*. Same patient in traction after plaster application. After plaster has set, one end of surcingle strap is divided and withdrawn from cast. Cast is then trimmed so that patient's head is free, and all edges are finished and windows are cut in cast to allow proper chest expansion. (Courtesy Stryker Corporation, Kalamazoo, Michigan.).

weeks of preoperative halofemoral traction, surgery is performed—with the patient in traction. Halofemoral traction is then resumed postoperatively for another 3 or more weeks. The patient is then put in a halo cast, which continues cephalopelvic distraction while he is ambulatory.

Halofemoral traction was modified during the past decade by DeWald, who devised a pelvic halo that is fixed to the patient's pelvis by long transfixion pins penetrating through the iliac wing on both sides. Extremely severe spinal deformities can be dramatically corrected with halo-hoop distraction, and respiratory function is undisturbed by encircling plaster casts (Fig. 11-10). Patients with severe pulmonary compromise can thus be adequately treated and ambulated at an early stage in their treatment white still maintaining dynamic corrective traction. The halo-hoop technique has been used with increasing efficiency in Hong Kong by Hodgson and Yau in treating patients with severe tuberculous and scoliotic spinal deformities. It has also been extremely helpful in the anterior approach surgery and cable technique of Dwyer.

In recent years, Cotrel has devised a form of traction that has proven to be most effective, especially in the preoperative treatment of patients with scoliosis and kyphosis. Soft rubber slings are criss-crossed around the pelvis and threaded to foot pedals that the patient can push. This exerts a distraction force between the pelvis and the head harness, which includes the patient's chin and occiput. Dramatic forces can thus be obtained with the patient in the supine position, and most forms of moderate scoliosis can be softened to permit preoperative ligamentous stretching with much better surgical results (Fig. 11-11). The Cotrel traction technique is most effective when it can be performed several weeks before surgery, but it is generally considered to be a presurgical adjunct and is not a substitute for surgery or bracing in the treatment of scoliosis.

Cotrel also devised the surgical "costotransversotomy." An osteotomy is performed directly through the transverse process of all the thoracic vertebrae on the convex side so that the rib hump can be adequately swung anteriorly to decrease the dorsal prominence of the convex ribs. Examination of the normal skeleton will reveal that the end of each rib articulates between two adjacent vertebral bodies. It then joins directly to the transverse process of the thoracic vertebrae and is held in position by the costotransverse ligaments. If an osteotomy is performed directly through the transverse processes of 6 to 8 ribs, the entire rib cage can be swung forward and hinged so that the rib deformity decreases (Fig. 11-12). This rib correction is then permanently held and enhanced by proper postoperative plaster technique and the rib deformities are permanently corrected after the plaster is removed.

The techniques used on the Scoliosis Service at the New York Orthopaedic Hospital consist of a thorough medical work-up, which involves an in-depth study of all bleeding and clotting factors. Pulmonary function is

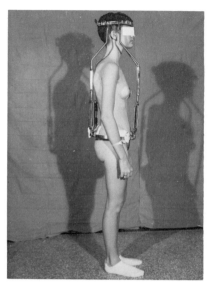

Fig. 11-10.   Halo-hoop traction devised by DeWald to correct spinal deformity without an encircling plaster cast. This technique's main advantage is that patients with severe respiratory deficit do not need to be encased in plaster, which further diminishes pulmonary function. Also, surgery can be performed in some instances while traction is maintained. Pelvic hoop is held in position by long transfixion pins that transverse iliac crests on both sides. (Courtesy Ronald L. DeWald, M.D.)

analyzed to detect any pulmonary deficit and determine whether such surgical adjuncts as tracheostomy will be necessary. New x-rays are then taken in both the erect and side-bending supine positions to determine curve flexibility and whether secondary curves are structural (Fig. 11-13). The lumbosacral articulation is examined for any anomaly such as spondylolisthesis or sacralization of the lowest lumbar segment.

Most adolescent girls who have reached menarche are placed on birth control pills to keep them from menstruating during surgery, since patients who are menstruating during surgery have increased blood loss due to clotting disturbances which have not been totally established as yet.

The selection of the fusion area is extremely important. In the routine patient with a thoracic or thoracolumbar curve, we generally fuse one vertebra above and two vertebrae below the major curve to be fused. If two curves are structural, they both need to be fused completely. One of the biggest mistakes in scoliosis surgery is making the spine fusion too short. Although we almost always avoid fusing to lumbar 5 or the sacrum, it is important to fuse all rotated

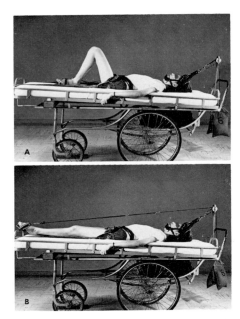

Fig. 11-11.   Cotrel traction using cervical halter and criss-cross
rubber pelvic straps that allow patient to control longitudinal spinal
traction by self-activated foot pedals. Technique allows progressive
stretching and softening of spinal ligaments and is preoperative
adjunct to scoliosis surgery. (Courtesy Professor Yves Cotrel.)

vertebrae, especially for single thoracic or thoracolumbar curves. Even though
the lower end vertebra may be T-12, if L-2 and 3 are severely rotated, they
should be included in the fusion area. Otherwise, the curve will extend after
the plaster has been removed, and the spine will be thrown out of balance.

If the patient has spondylolytic scoliosis, a simple fusion for spondylolisthesis causes the resulting scoliosis to correct by itself (Fig. 8-21). Then the
scoliosis need not be fused. However, if the spinal curve has been allowed to
become structural, it too must be fused or at least braced in aMilwaukee brace
until the patient is fully mature. Spondylolisthesis that is separate from the
scoliosis and is progressing or causing pain should be fused along with the
major scoliotic curve.

Sometimes one or two vertebrae can be skipped, such as in a right thoracic
curve where the fusion may extend to L-2, and then the facet joints for L-2, 3,
and 4 can be left open while the spondylolisthesis is fused from L-4 or 5 to the
sacrum (Fig. 11-14). Such combined cases can be performed at the same
surgical sitting with excellent end resutls. However, in all cases of spinal fusion
to the sacrum, one thigh should be included in the plaster cast to immobilize the

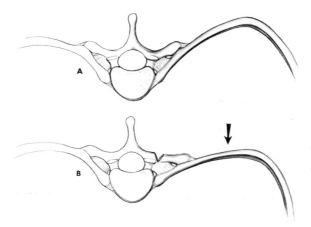

Fig. 11-12. Costotransversotomy to rib deformity on convex side. Normal rib articulates at its end between 2 adjacent thoracic vertebrae. Neck of rib touches transverse process and is held in place by costotransverse ligaments. If transverse process of thoracic vertebra is divided on convex side, entire rib can be angulated forward and deformity dramatically decreased. This must be done over a segment of 6 to 8 ribs on the convex side, and correction maintained by proper plaster technique using surcingle table and overhead Cotrel frame.

sacrum. This leg part of the cast should be maintained for at least 6 months after surgery, and some times when stress is marked in the lumbosacral area, the thigh portion should remain for the full 9 months after surgery.

If a patient has asymptomatic, nonprogressive spondylolisthesis, the spondylolisthesis should be ignored for the moment and surgery performed for the scoliosis alone. In young patients with progressive curves, it is much better to err on the side of too long a spinal fusion. Too short a fusion in immature patients with progressive scoliosis causes the spine to continue to curve, and the deformity progresses as these patients mature. However, in mature patients, the fusion can sometimes be slightly shorter than would normally be required because severe curve progression in an adult or late adolescent is generally unlikely after spinal fusion.

In recent years great interest has evolved in anterior spinal surgery. Dwyer pioneered the anterior approach and the application of a cable-bolt technique to correct severe spinal deformities. His technique has many advocates, but the approach—through a rib resection to the anterior spine—is more complicated than that used in posterior spinal surgery. The cable-bolt technique is excellent for patients with failed posterior surgery, posterior infections, or congenital defects such as myelomeningocele. It also dramatically corrects thoracolumbar and lumbar curves. It is contraindicated, however, in kyphosis, double struc-

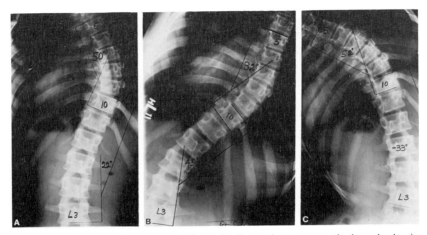

Fig. 11-13.   Side-bending x-rays aid in evaluating patient preoperatively and selecting proper fusion area. *A*. Patient has 50° right thoracic scoliosis and 22° left lumbar curve in erect film. *B* Patient is bent to right in supine x-ray and thoracic curve corrects to 32°, showing curve flexibility. But since curve has not corrected completely, it is a structural curve and must be fused in its entirety. *C*. Patient bends to left, increasing thoracic curve but markedly decreasing left lumbar curve to − 33°, which indicates that lumbar curve is flexible and does not need to be fused. Fusion from T-4 to T-12 produced excellent cosmetic and functional results.

tural scoliosis, very young patients, severely rigid curves, and thoracic scoliosis. Sometimes an anterior Dwyer technique and a posterior Harrington instrumentation can be combined to correct a complicated problem (Fig. 11-15).

After proper work-up, including good neurological and pediatric examinations, the patient is placed in a preoperative surcingle cast for 4 to 6 days. The preoperative cast has several functions. First, it conditions the patient to the plaster so that casting is not a traumatic experience postoperatively. Second, the dynamic forces of cast application stretch the soft tissue structures markedly. This permits even greater surgical correction. Third, the cast is split 2 days before surgery, and the posterior plaster shell is padded and used to splint the patient postoperatively until the final scoliosis cast is applied.

Surgery is performed directly through the cast at some medical centers with good results. However, we are greatly concerned with cardiac arrests during surgery and have found that having the patient out of plaster provides quick access to the thoracic region if a thoracotomy is required.

Finally, the application of the preoperative surcingle cast is helpful in that it stretches the patient's spine considerably, allowing the spinal cord to adjust to

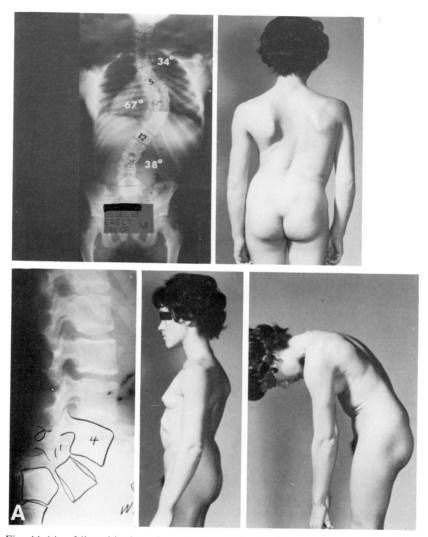

Fig. 11-14. Idiopathic thoracic scoliosis associated with severe symptomatic spondylolisthesis of L-5. *A*. Patient has marked cosmetic deformity and limited forward flexion because of hamstring muscle spasm secondary to spondylolisthesis. Scoliosis was corrected with fusion and Harrington instrumentation from T-5 to L-1. Lumbosacral level was fused 2 weeks later from L-3 to sacrum. *B*. Excellent functional and cosmetic results. (Reprinted with permission, Goldstein L A: Surgical management of scoliosis. Clin Orthop 17:46, 1971.)

179

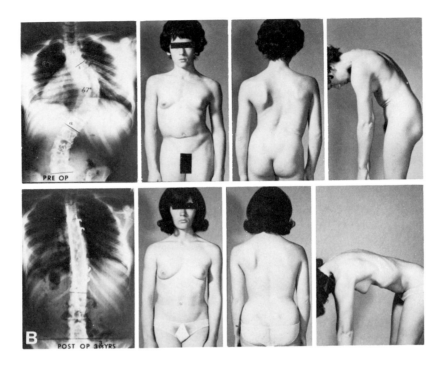

its new position inside the straightened neural canal. In patients with double major curves, actual standing height may sometimes be 6 or 8 cm shorter than corrected height after scoliosis surgery. Since the spinal cord has maintained a position conforming to the shortened neural canal for several years, a sudden corrective force such as that generated by instrumentation under anesthesia could produce a devastating, permanent neurological deficit.

Several of our patients who were placed in preoperative casts developed paresthesias and early paraplegia, which immediately improved when the cast was removed. Had these patients been brought to the hospital and given general anesthesia with internal instrumentation, the results could have been disastrous.

After the surcingle cast has been in place from 4 to 6 days, it is removed to allow skin care 2 days before surgery. At this time, adequate doses of prophylactic antibiotics are also given. We generally use sodium oxacillin in nonpenicillin allergic patients and other broad-spectrum antibiotics in patients with penicillin allergy. These antibiotics are continued during surgery and postoperatively for approximately 7 days. We have used prophylactic antibiotics for the past 6 years, and the incidence of wound infection has been

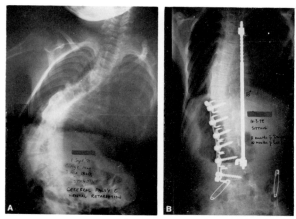

Fig. 11-15.   14-year, 11-month old child with cerebral palsy, mental retardation, severe thoracolumbar scoliosis, and marked pelvic obliquity. An anterior approach using Dwyer technique in lumbar region dramatically corrected lumbar curve and pelvic obliquity. Posterior spinal fusion using Harrington rod 1 month later produced this dramatic result. (Courtesy Robert B. Winter, M.D.)

practically eliminated and wound complications have decreased appreciably. Before we instituted prophylactic antibiotic therapy, the infection rate was approximately 5.75 percent.

At surgery, the patient is given a general inhalation anesthetic, and usually an indwelling Foley catheter is inserted so that urinary output can be monitored and situations such as blood incompatibility and transfusion reaction can be quickly observed by urinalysis or renal shutdown. We generally place the patient in an operative frame designed to hold him in the kneeling position, but with the buttocks inclined against the supporting seat so that the main areas of support are the knees, buttocks, and shoulders. The abdomen is completely free and lack of abdominal compression greatly reduces venous pressure in the portal circulation and bleeding during surgery (Fig. 11-16).

Routine hypotensive anesthesia includes halothane and occasional supplementary drugs to keep the systolic blood pressure near 75–80 mm Hg. The patient is extremely well monitored, many times using arterial catheters, especially in high risk patients, so that the blood gases can be easily ascertained during surgery, and all vital signs can be read on computer printouts.

The actual technique consists of a straight incision from the tip of the upper vertebra to the sacrum (Fig. 11-17A). The first incision is superficial, and the subcutaneous area is then injected with approximately 100 cc of 1:500,000 epinephrine-saline solution, which reduces local bleeding directly. The incision is then extended deeper using an electric scalpel, and the tips of the

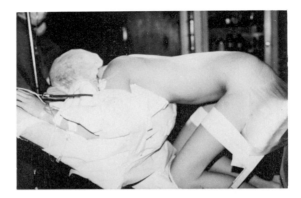

Fig. 11-16.   Spinal frame used for scoliosis surgery and also for lumbar spinal surgery in adults. Patient is in kneeling position and most weight is taken by buttocks resting on support behind upper thighs. A pillow placed directly beneath sternum eliminates thoracic lordosis, and entire abdomen is free. Operative table must be tilted so that spine parallels the floor. This operating frame, drastically reduces blood loss, and severe cases can be handled with excellent pulmonary ventilation. Over 500 scoliosis operations have been performed on this frame without complications.

spinous processes are localized and identified in their midline. Cobb elevators are then used to subperiosteally strip the soft tissue structures from the tips of the spinous processes. This is easy in young patients but becomes increasingly difficult in older patients.

The exact area in the spine must be localized, and this is easy when the fusion extends to L-3 or 4 since the exposure is merely carried down to the sacrum and an exact count from the sacrum can be made with little chance of error. Most patients have only one surgical incision, since the bone graft is removed through the same midline approach.

When the fusion is confined mainly to the thoracic region, a separate incision is made over the iliac crest in a vertical plane to avoid keloid scar formation over the iliac donor site. These areas are also infiltrated with dilute epinephrine solution in the paraspinal muscles to achieve more hemostasis.

Self-retaining retractors are used throughout to hold the muscle masses away from the midline, and if the approach has been made directly to the thoracic region, the 12th thoracic rib on one side of the spine is exposed, along with the transverse process of the uppermost lumbar vertebra. By using this technique, we have been much more accurate and have had much less difficulty than in obtaining a surgical x-ray to localize the exact vertebra.

After the proper end vertebrae are identified, a meticulous subperiosteal dissection is performed and all capsular and ligamentous structures are elevated from the vertebrae to be included in the fusion. Bleeding should be closely monitored during this phase and all bleeders cauterized to minimize blood loss.

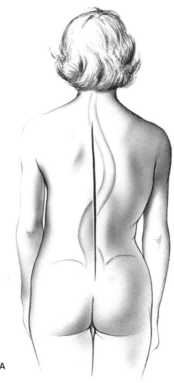

A

Fig. 11-17 *A*   Proper incision in posterior approach. Although spinal deformity is marked, incision is straight because when spine has been corrected incision will remain straight. This is more pleasing cosmetically and allows adequate exposure of underlying spinal elements. *B*. Diagram showing placement of 1252 Harrington hook at upper end of fusion site. Hook has been inserted into a previously cut notch in inferior aspect of thoracic vertebra chosen for hook. Blade is driven directly into pedicle of that vertebra and is gently impacted into place. *C*. Upper and lower Harrington hooks in place and Harrington outrigger inserted to distract spine. Amount of distraction should be judged carefully since all patients vary and no specific amount of traction can be advised for all patients. Younger patients are generally more flexible, and surgeon must not allow spinal cord to be overstretched. *D*. Harrington rod placement between upper and lower distraction hooks. Entire spine is then decorticated and autogenous cancellous and cortical bone placed directly along decorticated posterior spinal elements (upper end of figure). Lower end of figure has been shown without bone graft to illustrate thorough decortication and facet excision in lumbar region before adding bone graft.

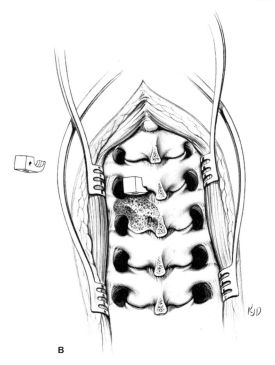

B

The upper Harrington hook is then inserted into a notch previously cut in the inferior facet area of the upper thoracic vertebra to be fused. This notch is cut using a ⅜-inch sharp osteotome, and it directly exposes the superior articular facet of the vertebra below the one in which the upper hook is then inserted. The most commonly used hook is the 1252 Harrington, which has a central keel and is locked directly into the pedicle by the blade of the hook and impacted gently into place for firm fixation (Fig. 11-17B). The lower Harrington hook, usually the 1254 hook, is inserted into a previously cut notch in the lamina of the lumbar vertebra chosen. After both the upper and lower hooks are in place, the Harrington outrigger is positioned and the spine is distracted (Fig. 11-17C). The outrigger is preferred because it stabilizes the spine and allows better decortication, and also because the exact Harrington rod to be used can be assessed accurately, eliminating guesswork.

With the spine in distraction, the wound is packed and attention focused on obtaining the autogenous iliac bone graft, which is usually approached through the same skin incision, but via a separate subcutaneous route directly over the iliac crest. The entire iliac crest is then stripped subperiosteally, and the Stryker impact osteotome is used to remove large amounts of cortical and cancellous

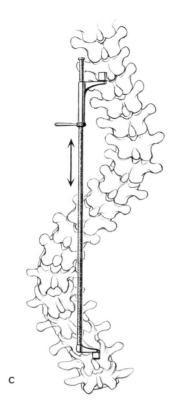

c

bone. This bone is cut into numerous small thin strips of graft material. As much bone as possible is removed from the iliac region, and the area is packed with small amounts of bone wax and gelfoam. The bone wax is impregnated directly into the cancellous iliac crest to reduce bleeding.

This area is then closed directly over a hemovac drain, and the posterior elements of all the vertebrae to be fused are decorticated. In the thoracic region, all posterior elements are widely decorticated with individual attention to the facet joints on the concave side. In the thoracolumbar and lumbar regions, all facet joints are destroyed. These joints are completely resected using the impact osteotome, so that bone graft material directly contacts the denuded vertebrae.

After decortication is complete, the bone graft that has been cut into numerous thin slivers is then impacted gently along the entire length of the fusion area. Once the graft is in place, the Harrington outrigger is removed and replaced with the proper Harrington rod, which is then distracted using the Harrington distractor to provide proper rod tension (Fig. 11-17D). A small

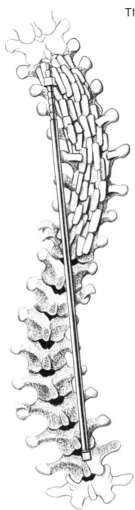

D

circle washer is then applied beneath the upper distraction hook to prevent hook slippage, hemovac tubes are inserted, and the wound is closed in layers.

A large compression dressing is then applied. The posterior plaster shell of the original preoperative cast is held on by an abdominal binder, and the patient is turned from the operating frame directly onto the recovery room cart and nursed in the posterior plaster shell for 8 to 10 days.

The first dressing change is generally made on the second day postoperatively, when most patients are free of their indwelling catheter and are beginning to take liquids orally. Antibiotics are continued for 7 to 9 days postoperatively, and at that time the sutures are removed and the final plaster cast is applied. Prophylactic gamma-globulin is given to all patients; this has reduced post-transfusion hepatitis statistically on our service. We generally give 5 cc of gamma-globulin in each buttock on the 5th and 8th days postoperatively.

Patients are ambulated immediately the day of final plaster application; their cast is trimmed and finished the next day, and they are then allowed to go home. Total hospital time usually does not exceed 19 or 20 days. Almost all patients resume normal activities, including a full course in school, approximately 3 weeks after they return home.

The plaster cast is not changed during the entire 9 months after surgery, mainly because the bone graft is making the greatest effort toward solid union at about the 5th to 7th months, and any attempt to remove the cast and apply a new corrective cast may cause a "green stick" fracture in the fusion mass, which may lead to nonunion and pseudoarthrosis. During these 9 months, however, the patient can be active and participate in minor sports, such as bowling or tennis. Obviously, the sooner patients return to original friends and activities, the sooner they improve psychologically and the less difficulty they have in adjusting to their usual routine.

With the aforementioned technique, the correction of most types of scoliotic spine deformities has been uniformly rewarding at the New York Orthopaedic Hospital. In patients who have congenital scoliosis or severely deformed and structural curves, other techniques—such as spinal osteotomy, halofemoral traction, or anterior surgical approaches—are often necessary. Sometimes a combination of procedures and techniques spaced at various intervals is desirable, and each of these must be chosen to fit the patient.

In general, scoliosis surgery is a major and metabolically traumatic operation. It should not be performed by an inexperienced or "occasional" surgeon since many pitfalls can arise with disastrous complications. However, scoliosis surgery performed by a skilled technician in a modern hospital setting with a team of experts can have extremely rewarding and dramatic functional results.

ELECTROSPINAL INSTRUMENTATION

Electrical energy has long been considered as a potential tool in treating scoliosis. But it was not until 1969 that Bobechko of the Hospital for Sick Children in Toronto began animal experiments showing that scoliosis could be produced electrically. Together with Herbert, a research biophysicist, who devised much of the initial electronic circuitry used in experimental animals, Bobechko continued the research.

At first young pigs were made scoliotic by placing electrodes on one side of a normally straight spine. The painless electrical impulses gradually produced scoliosis over the next few weeks. Scoliosis could then be reduced and

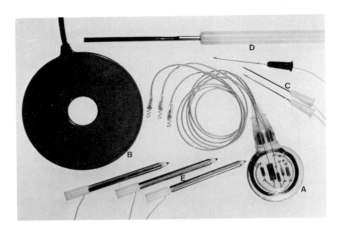

Fig. 11-18. Instruments used in electrospinal instrumentation. *A*. Radio receiver is implanted in subcutaneous tissue next to spine; 3 "corkscrew" electrodes anchor into selected muscle sites. *B*. External antenna picks up signals from radio transmitter the patient wears. *C*. Original "needle electrodes" to determine proper site for electrode placement. *D*. Tool for inserting corkscrew electrodes. *E*. "Probe electrodes" are inserted after needle electrodes and before final placement of corkscrew electrodes. (Courtesy Medtronic Inc., Minneapolis, Minnesota.)

even reversed by placing the stimulating electrodes on the opposite (or convex) side of the scoliotic curve.

Friedman, a biomedical engineer representing Medtronic, Inc., of Minneapolis, joined the group in 1972 and helped greatly in designing and developing a complete system to correct scoliosis in humans (Fig. 11-18).

The first human implant was carried out by the Toronto team in February 1973. Encouraged by their early results, the research group was expanded to include the author, who was aided by Robert Pawluk, a research physicist, and Dr. Newton C. McCollough of Miami. The objective of these three clinical research groups was to evaluate electrospinal instrumentation on selected patients. At first, mainly right thoracic curves in girls with flexible spines and bone ages of 13 or 14 were selected for correction.

By March 1975, Bobechko and his team had already implanted 18 electrospinal units, and early results were encouraging. The first electrospinal instrumentations (ESI) in the United States were performed in May 1975, first at the New York Orthopaedic Hospital and then at the Jackson Memorial Hospital of the University of Miami (Fig. 11-19).

Although this type of work is still experimental, it shows promise of new avenues and goals to be reached in the correction of the scoliotic spine. Hopefully, future applications using high-energy sources and other sophisticated means of scoliosis treatment will make the management of scoliosis easier and more successful than in the past.

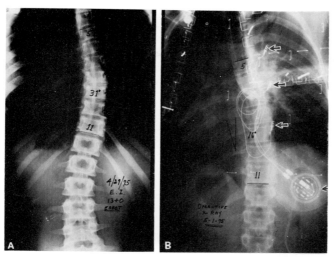

Fig. 11-19.   13-year-old girl with 31° right thoracic scoliosis from T-5 to T-11 who
was flexible on side-bending. Electrospinal instrumentation was performed on May 1,
1975. B. Patient is on operating frame with electrospinal implant inserted. Supine
scoliosis was 22°, but on direct impulse from power source, spinal muscles contracted
on convex side at site of 3 corkscrew electrodes *(small arrows)*, and scoliosis was
corrected to 16°. Radio receiver and overlying external antenna are in lower right corner
(arrow).

REFERENCES

1. Apley AG: Transthoracic approach in the treatment of scoliosis. Proc R Soc Med
    54:281, 1961
2. Cotrel Y, Morel G: La technique de l'E.D.F. dans la correction des scoliosis. Rev
    Chir Orthop 50:59, 1964
3. DeWald R, Ray RD: Skeletal traction for the treatment of severe scoliosis. J Bone
    Joint Surg 53A:233, 1970
4. DiStefano VJ, Klein KS, Nixon JE, et al: Intraoperative analysis of the effects of
    position and body habitus on surgery of the low back. Clin Orthop 99:51–56, 1974
5. Dolan JA, MacEwen GD: Surgical treatment of scoliosis. Clin Orthop 76:125,
    1971
6. Dwyer AF: Experience of anterior correction of scoliosis. Clin Orthop
    93:191–206, 1973
7. Dwyer AF, Newton NC, Sherwood AA: An anterior approach to scoliosis. Clin
    Orthop 62:192, 1969
8. Evarts CM, Winter RB, Hall JE: Vascular compression of the duodenum as-
    sociated with the treatment of scoliosis. Review of the literature and report of 18
    cases. J Bone Joint Surg 53A:431–444, 1971

9. Goldstein LA: Treatment of idiopathic scoliosis by Harrington instrumentation and fusion with fresh autogenous iliac bone grafts. Results in 80 patients. J Bone Joint Surg 51A:209, 1969

10. Goldstein LA: The surgical treatment of idiopathic scoliosis. Clin Orthop 93:131–157, 1973

11. Goldstein LA: The surgical management of scoliosis. Clin Orthop 77:32, 1971

12. Goldstein LA: Rib Resection and Concave Ligament Release and the Correction of Idiopathic Thoracic Scoliosis. American Academy of Orthopaedic Surgeons, Symposium on the Spine. St. Louis, Mosby, 1969

13. Gruca A: Surgical treatment of scoliosis in children, in Chapchal G (ed): Operative Treatment of Scoliosis. New York, Intercontinental Medical Book, 1973, p 108

14. Hall JE: Idiopathic scoliosis, indications for treatment, and follow-up study of 210 cases treated by Harrington instrumentation, in Keim H (ed): Second Annual Post-Graduate Course on the Management and Care of the Scoliosis Patient. Warsaw, Indiana, Zimmer, 1970, pp 23–26

15. Hardy JH, Takahashi RM, Peterson CA: Results of early ambulation following scoliosis spine fusion and Harrington rodding. J Bone Joint Surg 55A:436, 1973

16. Harrington PR: Technical details in relation to the successful use of instrumentation in scoliosis. Orthop Clin North Am 3:1, 49, 1972

17. Harrington PR: The history and development of Harrington instrumentation. Clin Orthop 93:110–130, 1970

18. Harrington PR: Treatment of scoliosis. Correction and internal fixation by spine instrumentation. J Bone Joint Surg 44A:591, 1962

19. Harrington PR, Dickson JH: An eleven-year clinical investigation of Harrington instrumentation: a preliminary report on 578 cases. Clin Orthop 93:82, 1973

20. Kastuik JP, Israel J, Hall JE: Scoliosis surgery in adults. Clin Orthop 93:225–234, 1973

21. Leatherman KD: The management of rigid spinal curves. Clin Orthop 93:215–224, 1973

22. Leider L, Moe J, Winter RB: Early ambulation after the surgical treatment of idiopathic scoliosis. Paper presented at American Orthopaedic Association meeting, Bermuda, June, 1972 (to be published)

23. MacKay IM: A new frame for the positioning of patients for surgery of the back. Can Anaesth Soc J 3:279, 1956

24. Moe JH: A critical analysis of methods of fusion for scoliosis. An evaluation in 266 patients. J Bone Joint Surg, 40A:529, 1958

25. Moe JH:Methods and Techniques of Evaluation of Idiopathic Scoliosis. American Academy of Orthopaedic Surgeons, Symposium on the Spine. St. Louis, Mosby, 1969

26. Morgenstern M, Hassmann, GC, Keim HA:Modifying post-transfusion hepatitis by gamma globulin in spinal surgery. Orthop Rev 4 6:29–32, 1975

27. Nachemson A: A long-term follow-up study of non-treated scoliosis. Acta Orthop Scand 30:446, 1968

28. O'Brien JP, Yau AC, Hodgson AR: Halo-pelvic traction: a technic for severe spinal deformities. Clin Orthop 93:179–190, 1973

29. Relton JES, Hall JE: Reduction of hemorrhage during spinal fusion combined with internal metallic fixation using a new scoliosis operating frame. J Bone Joint Surg 49B:327, 1967
30. Riseborough EJ: The anterior approach to the spine for the correction of deformities of the axial skeleton. Clin Orthop 93:207–214, 1973
31. Shannon DC, Riseborough EJ, Kazemi H: Ventilation perfusion relationship following correction of kyphoscoliosis. J Bone Joint Surg 53A:195, 1971
32. Siegel IM: Scoliosis in muscular dystrophy. Clin Orthop 93:235–238, 1973
33. Vauzelle C, Stagnara P, Jouvinroux P: Functional monitoring of spinal cord activity during spinal surgery. Clin Orthop 93:173–178, 1973

12
Kyphosis and Lordosis

CLASSIFICATION AND TREATMENT

Kyphosis is a change in the alignment of the spine in a sagittal plane that increases the posterior convex angulation. Normally, there is a thoracic kyphos measuring between 20° and 40° by the Cobb technique. During embryonic development, the entire spine has a kyphotic shape; but shortly after birth, the normal cervical and lumbar lordosis develops, allowing the head to be over the pelvis in the coronal plane.

Hall and Winter have classified kyphosis into 13 major groups (Table 12-1).

Postural

The first and most common type of kyphosis is postural kyphosis. This is not a directly pathological condition but seems to be part of the adolescent posture that is becoming all too common. Children assume bizarre sitting and standing attitudes that aggravate their postural kyphosis, especially during the adolescent growth spurt, unless remedial measures are taken. Postural kyphosis is especially common in an adolescent girl because breast development sometimes makes her extremely self-conscious. She assumes a round-shouldered slouch in order to hide her breasts, especially if she is tall for her age.

Sometimes this slouching is due to religious inhibitions of the parents or the child, and counseling the child to appreciate what God has created often

Table 12-1
Classification of Kyphosis

I.   Postural
II.   Scheuermann's
III. Congenital
      A.   Failure of formation
      B.   Failure of segmentation
      C.   Mixed
IV.   Paralytic
      A.   Polio
      B.   Anterior horn cell disease
      C.   Upper motor neuron disease (e.g., cerebral palsy)
V.   Myelomeningocele
VI.   Post-traumatic
      A.   Acute
      B.   Chronic
      C.   With or without cord damage
VII. Inflammatory
      A.   Tuberculosis
      B.   Other infection
VIII. Postsurgical
      A.   Postlaminectomy
      B.   After body excision (e.g., tumor)
IX.   Postirradiation
      A.   Neuroblastoma
      B.   Wilms' tumor
X.   Metabolic
      A.   Osteoporosis
           1.   Senile
           2.   Juvenile
      B.   Osteogenesis imperfecta
XI.   Developmental
      A.   Achondroplasia
      B.   Mucopolysaccharidoses
      C.   Other
XII. Collagen disease (e.g., Marie-Strümpell)
XIII. Tumor (e.g., histiocytosis X)

encourages her to walk erect and with her shoulders back. Aside from this, the general treatment of postural kyphosis is an exercise program and education in proper sitting and standing. On rare occasions, a Milwaukee brace is necessary (Fig. 12-1). Prompt remission with bracing is usually the rule since structural abnormalities are rare, and most of these children respond beautifully when given encouragement and exercise along with brace treatment.

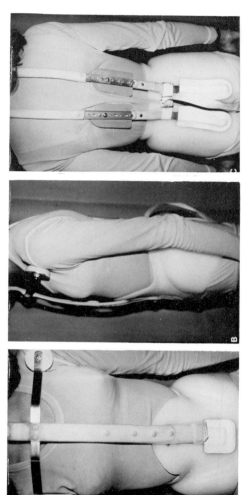

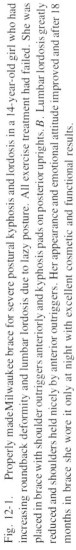

Fig. 12-1. Properly made Milwaukee brace for severe postural kyphosis and lordosis in a 14-year-old girl who had increasing roundback deformity and lumbar lordosis due to lazy posture. All exercise treatment had failed. She was placed in brace with shoulder outriggers anteriorly and kyphosis pads on posterior uprights. *B*. Lumbar lordosis greatly reduced and shoulders held nicely by anterior outriggers. Her appearance and emotional attitude improved and after 18 months in brace she wore it only at night with excellent cosmetic and functional results.

195

Scheuermann's Kyphosis

Scheuermann's kyphosis is an arcuate and fixed kyphosis developing at puberty. It is caused by a wedge-shaped deformity of usually 3 to 5 vertebrae with specific x-ray changes. The characteristic anterior wedging of the vertebral bodies with diminished anterior height was first described in 1920 by Scheuermann, who made it clear that the condition could be diagnosed definitely only after x-ray examination. The roentgenographic definition of Scheuermann's kyphosis is a kyphos including at least 3 adjacent vertebrae with wedging of 5° or more in each vertebra (Fig. 12-2).

The etiology of Scheuermann's kyphosis is unknown; however, hundreds of theories have been proposed. Scheuermann postulated that avascular necrosis of the cartilage ring apophysis of the vertebral body caused the disease process. Bick and Copel noted in 1951 that the ring apophysis was not connected to the growth plate and could not contribute to the longitudinal growth of the vertebrae; therefore, any changes in the apophysis or limbus did not alter the growth potential of the vertebral body.

Schmorl noted in 1931 that intervertebral disc material could herniate through the growth plate and produce kyphosis. To substantiate his views, Schmorl performed autopsies on 6 patients between the ages of 16 and 24 with Scheuermann's kyphosis. His theory was challenged, however, by the finding that such changes in the vertebrae outside the area of kyphosis occurred in patients with Scheuermann's disease and even in persons with perfectly normal spines.

Mechanical forces have also been implicated along with changes in the vascular supply through the anterior groove of the vertebral body. The theory of mechanical injury as a cause does not have an experimental basis, and the incidence of Scheuermann's disease in children involved in heavy manual labor is no higher than in other children. Bradford et al have postulated that Scheuermann's kyphosis may be a form of juvenile osteoporosis. They studied 12 patients with this condition and noted increased bone resorption in 5; dietary analysis suggested calcium deficiency as an etiological important factor. The incidence of Scheuermann's kyphosis is increased in nontropical sprue, Turner's syndrome, and cystic fibrosis.

The incidence of Scheuermann's disease has been reported between 0.5 and 8 percent of the general population. It seems to affect males and females equally; however, in Bradford's series the female to male ratio was 2 to 1. The exact age of onset of the condition is difficult to determine because x-ray changes typical of Scheuermann's kyphosis are generally not seen before age 11.

The typical patient is usually between 13 and 17 years old and complains of poor posture, fatigue, and/or pain near the kyphos. The back pain is usually aggravated by lengthy standing in the same position and is relieved by lying

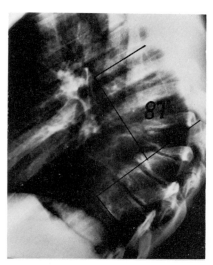

Fig. 12-2.   Scheuermann's kyphosis with marked wedge-shaped
formation of middle thoracic vertebrae and 87° kyphosis. Vertebral
bodies have moth-eaten appearance along anteroinferior borders.

down. The kyphosis is purely thoracic in about 75 percent of patients and
thoracolumbar in the other 25 percent. Lumbar lordisis is increased and the
abdomen is prominent. The trunk is held backward so that the center of gravity
falls behind the sacrum, and normal pelvic tilt is exaggerated. The increased
cervical and lumbar lordosis is a compensatory mechanism (Fig. 12-3). Mild
scoliosis is present in 30 to 40 percent of patients with Scheuermann's
kyphosis.

The patient usually has local tenderness, especially upon attempts to
correct the deformity, and in severe cases there are neurological findings of
spinal cord compression. The hamstrings are usually shortened, and the patient
cannot touch the floor by bending forward.

The vertebral body wedging is most marked in the central area of the
kyphosis. The "kyphotic angle" is the angle measured from lines drawn from
the superior border of the upper end vertebra and the inferior border of the lower
end vertebra, with perpendicular lines drawn from the end vertebrae lines to
measure the intersecting angle, as in the Cobb technique for measuring
scoliosis. A measurement over 40° is generally considered abnormal. The early
x-ray findings of Scheuermann's disease are wedging, Schmorl's nodes, and
irregular end plates. Late x-ray changes show progressive end plate irregularity
with severe vertebral wedging in advanced cases. Mau has classified the natural
course of Scheuermann's kyphosis in four roentgenographic stages: (1) irritation; (2) deformation with the development of wedging; (3) repair; and (4)
proliferation. During the last two stages, the vertebral end plates narrow

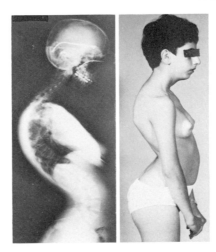

Fig. 12-3.   Scheuermann's disease in adolescent girl with severe
thoracic kyphosis and associated lumbar lordosis. Her appearance
was unacceptable. Cases of this sort almost never respond to exercise programs and generally need aggressive spinal Milwaukee
bracing. Sometimes recalcitrant curves need surgery for optimum
correction. (Courtesy Louis A. Goldstein, M.D.)

severely and osteophytes form, leading to arthritic changes in adult life and
increasing back pain.

In mild forms, Scheuermann's disease can generally be treated by exercises
and, if pain is severe, short periods of casting. Exercises alone are rarely of
much benefit but when coupled with theMilwaukee brace can be most helpful.
TheMilwaukee brace treatment, originally described by Blount in 1958, is the
most effective therapy for Scheuermann's kyphosis (Fig. 12-4). Often combined methods of treatment—bed rest, traction, plaster casting, and bracing-
—can produce a good end result.

Bradford et al. recently reviewed 223 patients with Scheuermann's
kyphosis and postural roundback. Kyphosis was improved by an average of 40
percent in 75 of their patients who had completed Milwaukee brace treatment.
The vertebral wedging was improved by an average of 41 percent and lordosis
improved by 46 percent. Factors that limited the amount of correction with the
Milwaukee brace were kyphotic curves greater than 65°, skeletal maturity of the
patient, and vertebral wedging greater than 10° per vertebra.

Some patients who do not respond toMilwaukee bracing or have advanced
curves and severe back pain need to have surgical correction. This is best done
from a posterior approach in moderate cases, using bilateral Harrington compression instruments and spinal fusion. In severe cases, both an anterior
approach with rib strut grafts and a second-stage posterior approach may be
necessary (Fig. 12-5).

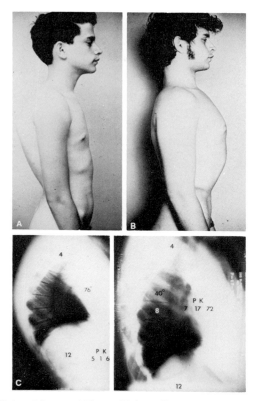

Fig. 12-4.   16-year-old boy with juvenile roundback secondary to
Scheuermann's disease. He had a bone age of slightly over 14
years, and Milwaukee bracing was used to reduce kyphotic deformity from 76° to 40° *(C)*. *B*. Excellent posture and good end result 4
years after treatment. (Courtesy Walter P. Blount, M.D.)

Congenital

Congenital kyphosis, mentioned in Chapter 1, is further divided into three
subgroups: (1) failure of formation anteriorly, in which all or part of a vertebral
body is absent (Fig. 12-6A); (2) failure of segmentation anteriorly, in which
there is an anterior unsegmented bar (Fig. 12-6B); and (3) mixed types in which
types 1 and 2 are combined.

Winter, Moe, and Wang studied the histories of 130 patients with
kyphosis. All three types were seen in all sites in the spine, but paraplegia
occurred only in unstable type 1 lesions (6 of 24 untreated cases). Without
treatment, regular progression of the kyphosis was the rule and averaged 7° per
year, reaching maximum progression during the adolescent growth spurt.

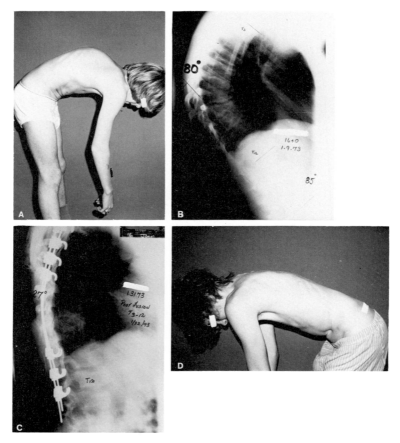

Fig. 12-5.   16-year-old boy with increasing back pain and severe kyphotic deformity
secondary to Scheuermann's disease. Anterior thoracic approach using rib strut grafts to
prop up vertebral bodies was followed by posterior spinal fusion using 2 sets of
Harrington-type compression instruments *(C)*. *D*. Postoperative correction on forward
bending. Cosmetic and functional results were good. (Courtesy David S. Bradford,
M.D.)

Brace treatment was ineffective and 44 patients required surgery. Pseudoarthrosis in posterior fusions occurred in 15 of 28 patients, but in only 2 of 16
patients who had anterior and posterior spine fusions. Correction with posterior
fusion before the age of 3 is recommended treatment; however, in cases with
angulation over 50°, the combined posterior and anterior spine fusions are
recommended. In almost all children, congenital kyphosis
progressed-significantly. Severe deformity leading to paraplegia was quite
common, and even qualified orthopedic surgeons tend to be unaware of the
severely malignant capabilities of this condition.

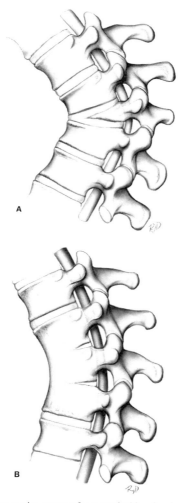

Fig. 12-6. Two major types of congenital kyphosis. *A*. Failure of formation of vertebral element. Vertebral body is small and deformed, and posterior element is rudimentary. Sometimes 3 or 4 vertebral bodies are absent, resulting in severe kyphotic deformity. *B*. Failure of segmentation causes an unsegmented congenital bar anteriorly. Resultant tethering mechanism leads to increasing kyphosis due to continued posterior spinal bone growth.

In certain advanced cases, anterior osteotomy of the vertebral bodies is necessary to preserve spinal formation and correct the deformity. Such techniques are extremely hazardous and should be performed only by spinal surgeons specifically trained in this work. Postoperative management generally is 1 year of cast immobilization with the first 6 months being spent in bed. The rapidly growing spines of children should be protected with a Milwaukee brace after their cast is removed and until spinal growth is complete. In cases of paraplegia due to congenital kyphosis, never allow a laminectomy to be performed because the spinal cord is stretched tightly over the vertebral bodies in front, and laminectomy only removes valuable bone and ligaments, usually leading to increasing deformity and more spinal cord compression.

The treatment of progressive nerve deficit in congenital kyphosis is decompression of the spinal cord anteriorly through the posterior longitudinal ligament to allow the spinal cord and dura to move anteriorly in the surgically created cavity and to decompress the spinal cord. An anterior strut spine fusion is always necessary at this time (Fig. 12-7).

The most important rule in congenital kyphosis and scoliosis is to *never allow progression*. If an astute combination of casting, bracing, and surgery is followed until the patient is fully mature, excellent results can be expected. Unfortunately, congenital kyphosis is only ¼ as common as congenital scoliosis but has a complication rate 4 times greater. Therefore, early diagnosis and treatment in congenital kyphosis are imperative.

Paralytic

Paralytic kyphosis is usually due to polio, anterior horn cell disease, or an upper motor neuron lesion such as cerebral palsy. These conditions usually can be well treated by spinal bracing in the early stages, but occasionally surgical maneuvers are necessary to obtain a good end result. When paralysis is secondary to kyphosis, all forms of corrective traction (such as halofemoral traction) are contraindicated because they can cause the already compressed spinal cord to be stretched even more over the apex of the kyphos, leading to greater spinal cord compression.

MYELOMENINGOCELE

Myelomeningocele kyphosis can be extremely severe because affected children are born without stabilizing posterior spinal elements. Previously, most of these children died at an early age; but with new techniques of prompt surgical closure of the spinal defect and antibiotics, many of them live to advanced adult life, sometimes with severe spinal deformities. In a recent study

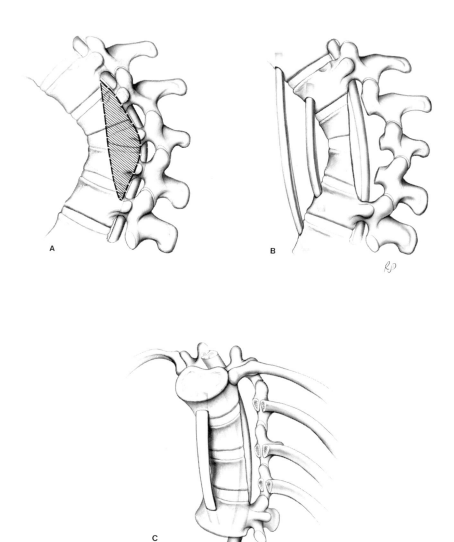

Fig. 12-7. Technique of anterior decompression of paraplegia due to congenital kyphosis. *A*. Spinal cord is compressed due to increasing congenital deformity. Vertebral bodies just anterior to posterior longitudinal ligament must be completely removed as well as ligament itself. *B*. Spinal cord is moved anteriorly after posterior longitudinal ligament has been released to allow proper spinal cord decompression. Never perform a laminectomy in cases of kyphotic deformity since this only increases problem by removing stabilizing elements posteriorly. *C*. Rib strut grafting from in front to prop up corrected vertebral bodies and reduce kyphosis. Posterior spinal fusion is sometimes necessary as a second stage to anterior strut grafting and decompression.

203

by Hall et al, 130 patients were followed to age 18 and older. Of these, 101 developed significant spinal deformities. Therefore, 70 to 80 percent of patients with myelomeningocele probably will develop severe spinal deformities (usually scoliosis and kyphosis) by age 18.

Myelomeningocele kyphosis is usually present at birth and is probably the most difficult of all spinal conditions to treat. The patients are almost always paralyzed below the level of thoracic 12, and often they have associated anomalies of the cardiovascular and urinary systems. Patients are best managed by a combination of casting, bracing, and anterior spinal surgery. Good results are almost impossible to obtain with a posterior spine fusion because of the lack of good bone in that region. Patients with myelomeningocele kyphosis must be treated aggressively, and their condition must not be allowed to progress.

Post-traumatic

Post-traumatic kyphosis can be acute or chronic and may or may not be associated with spinal cord damage. This deformity was discussed in detail in the chapter on trauma (Chapter 6); commonly it results from high-speed automobile accidents with rapid deceleration. Post-traumatic kyphosis should be treated promptly with spinal traction. Cases of spinal cord damage with a progressing lesion should be treated with an anterior spinal cord decompression and never a *posterior* laminectomy since this increases both spinal instability and the deformity. (Fig. 6-6).

Inflammatory

Inflammatory kyphosis is almost always due to tuberculosis but can occur with other forms of osteomyelitis. This condition, discussed in the chapter on infections (Chapter 7), can usually be managed best in tuberculosis with spinal cord compression by an anterior decompression and spine fusion followed in some instances by a posterior fusion.

Postsurgical

Kyphosis following surgery is unfortunately far too common after an ill-advised laminectomy. Orthopedic surgeons must constantly state that laminectomy, in most forms of trauma and congenital kyphosis, almost always aggravates spinal cord compression. Occasionally, posterior vertebral resection of a tumor is necessary, and this renders the spine unstable and leads to progressing kyphosis. In these instances, tumor surgery should be followed with a second-stage posterior spine fusion. If this is not possible, an anterior fusion should be performed.

Postirradiation

Postirridation kyphosis is seen less frequently now that we have better x-ray control and understanding of the condition than years ago. It is most common following irradiation in infants for neuroblastoma or Wilms' tumor (Fig. 8-19). When it is obvious that such essential irradiation for tumor cure has caused epiphyseal damage and arrested growth in the spine, prompt spinal fusion should be performed to prevent increasing deformity.

Metabolic

Some metabolic conditions can lead to adolescent kyphosis. Osteoporosis, tropical diseases (such as sprue), and osteogenesis imprefecta can cause progressive kyphosis and are managed by treating the underlying disease and applying proper spinal bracing until the patient is mature.

Developmental

Developmental conditions, such as the various forms of dwarfism, must be treated individually. Morquio dwarfs especially tend to become severely kyphotic. They can be helped by judicious spinal bracing during their early adolescent years (Fig. 12-8).

Collagen Disease

Collagen disease occasionally leads to progressing kyphosis, especially in the adult. Marie-Strümpell arthritis causes severely progressing thoracic kyphosis. Affected patients sometimes develop such severe deformities in adult life that they cannot see where they are walking. In advanced cases, multiple spinal osteotomies are performed and the patient's spine is corrected to acceptable limits.

Tumor

Certain tumors, notably eosinophilic granuloma of the histiocytosis X type, lead to progressing kyphosis. This condition usually resolves spontaneously after maturation, and disc space height almost always resumes its normal configuration (Fig. 5-6). Milwaukee bracing may become necessary during

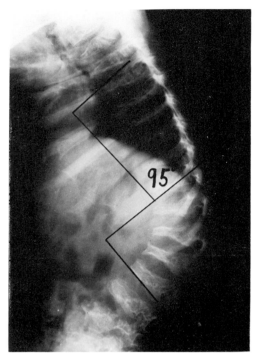

Fig. 12-8.   Progressive kyphosis in a metatrophic dwarf. 95°
kyphosis is due to uniform osteoporosis and wedge-shaped formation of all vertebral bodies in thoracic and lumbar spine.

active stages of this condition (Fig. 12-9). Neurofibromatosis is a hereditary
skeletal dysplasia (described in Chapter 5) that often leads to severe kyphotic
deformities, which can rapidly result in paraplegia if untreated (Fig. 12-10).

Lordosis

A normal lumbar lordosis is essential to compensate for thoracic kyphosis.
However, in some instances patients develop increasing lumbar lordosis that
can cause severely progressive low back pain in adult life. Although most
forms of excessive lordosis are postural, some forms of lordosis are secondary
to such conditions as myelomeningocele, dwarfism, retroperitoneal shunts for
hydrocephaly, spondylolisthesis, and trauma. Specific treatments of each of
these conditions usually reduces the lumbar lordosis to acceptable limits;
however, spine fusion is often necessary to achieve this.

Mild postural lordosis can be treated effectively by proper exercises and

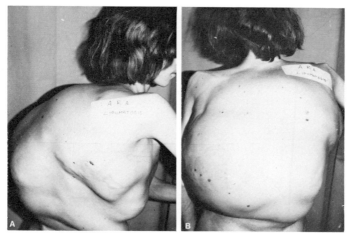

Fig. 12-9. Severe kyphotic deformity in a 12-year-old boy with generalized lipomatosis of axial skeleton. A previous attempt at tumor resection resulted in severe uncontrollable hemorrhage and left remainder of tumor unresectable. Patient became completely paraplegic 1 month after these photos were taken.

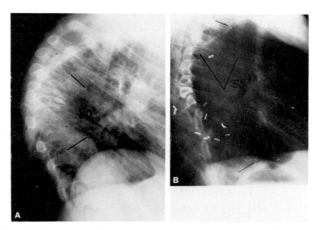

Fig. 12-10. Neurofibromatosis leading to progressive kyphotic deformity (same patient as in Fig. 5-11) of 80° in thoracic spine. Spine involved with neurofibromatosis has waferlife appearance. Anterior approach was made and rib strut grafts inserted in front to correct kyphosis from 80° to 55°. Second stage posterior spine fusion produced good cosmetic and functional results.

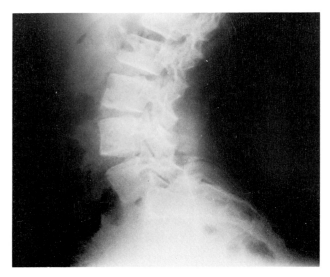

Fig. 12-11.   Postural lordosis in a 14-year-old girl who also had
associated roundback. Proper abdominal exercises and instruction
in pelvic tilt corrected deformity, and spinal bracing was unneces-
sary.

strengthening of the abdominal musculature (Fig. 12-11).Milwaukee bracing is
extremely effective in reducing excessive lumbar lordosis, and when properly
applied and maintained to maturity, braces can give permanent results.

REFERENCES

1. Blount WP,Moe JH: TheMilwaukee Brace. Baltimore, Williams & Wilkins, 1973
2. Bradford DS,Moe JH, Winter RB: Scoliosis, in Rothman RH, Simeone FA (eds):
    The Spine, vol. I. Philadelphia, Saunders, 1975, pp 271–380
3. Bradford DS,Moe JH,Montalvo E, et al: Scheuermann's kyphosis and roundback
    deformity—results of Milwaukee brace treatment. J Bone Joint Surg
    56A:740–758, 1954
4. Bradford DS: Neurological complications in Scheuermann's disease. J Bone Joint
    Surg 51A:567–572, 1969
5. Bunch WH: in Bunch WH, Cassl AS, Bernsman AS, Long DM (eds): Modern
    Management of Myelomeningocoele. St. Louis, 1972, pp 121–167
6. Dameron TB, Gulledge WH: Adolescent kyphosis. U S Armed Forces Med J
    4:871–875, 1953
7. Ferguson AB Jr: Etiology of pre-adolescent kyphosis. J Bone Joint Surg
    38A:149–157, 1956
8. Hafner RH: Localized osteochondritis. Scheuermann's disease. J Bone Joint Surg
    34B:38–40, 1952

9. James JIP: Kyphoscoliosis. J Bone Joint Surg 37B:414–426, 1955
10. Kemp FH, Wilson DC: Social and nutritional factors in adolescent osteochondritis of the spine. Br J Soc Med 2:66–70, 1948
11. Kemp FH, Wilson DC: A further report on factors in the etiology of osteochondritis of the spine. Br J Radiol 21:449–451, 1948
12. Knutson F: Observations on the growth of the vertebral body in Scheuermann's disease. Acta Radiol 30:97–104, 1948
13. Lambrinudi L: Adolescent and senile kyphosis. Br Med J 2:800–804, 1934
14. Michell AA: Osteochondrosis deformans juvenilis dorsi. NY State J Med 61:98–101, 1961
15. Moe JH: Treatment of adolescent kyphosis by nonoperative and operative methods. Manitoba Med Rev 45:481–484, 1965
16. Outland T, Snedden HE: Juvenile dorsal kyphosis. Clin Orthop 5:155–163, 1955
17. Overgaard K: Prolapses of nucleus pulposus and Scheuermann's disease. Nord Med 5:593–603, 1940
18. Scheuermann HW: Kyfosis dorsalis juvenilis. Ugesk Raeger 82:385–393, 1920
19. Schmorl G, Junghanns R: The Human Spine in Health and Disease. New York, Grune & Stratton, 1971
20. Simon RS: Diagnosis and treatment of kyphosis dorsalis juvenilis in early stage. J Bone Joint Surg 24:681–683, 1942
21. Sorensen KH: Scheuermann's Juvenile Kyphosis. Copenhagen, Munksgaard, 1964
22. Wassman K: Kyphosis juvenilis Scheuerman. Acta Orthop Scand 21:65–74, 1951
23. Winter RB, Moe JH, Wang JF: Congenital kyphosis, its natural history and treatment as observed in a study of 130 patients. J Bone Joint Surg 55A:223–256, 1973

Index